Neuroradiology in Clinical Practice

Abdul Qayyum Rana
Lawrence A. Zumo • Valerie Sim

Neuroradiology
in Clinical Practice

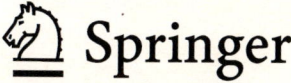 Springer

Abdul Qayyum Rana
Parkinson's Clinic
of Eastern Toronto
Toronto
ON
Canada

Lawrence A. Zumo
Silver Spring
Cheverly
MD
USA

Valerie Sim
Centre for Prions and Protein
Folding Diseases
University of Alberta
Edmonton
AB
Canada

ISBN 978-3-319-01001-4   ISBN 978-3-319-01002-1   (eBook)
DOI 10.1007/978-3-319-01002-1
Springer Cham Heidelberg New York Dordrecht London

Library of Congress Control Number: 2013945858

Printed on acid-free paper

Springer is part of Springer Science+Business Media (www.springer.com)

*To Kesselly, Malaika, Abdullah, Ruqqiyah,
Muhammad, Safwaan, Zainaab, and Ahmad, all
who had to endure mandatory time off whilst
the atlas was being prepared and to our beloved
spouses, Afshan, Janet, and Dominik, without
whose patient support the timely completion of this
work would not have been possible.*

Preface

This book is designed to provide a review of imaging characteristics of major neurological conditions for medical students during their neurology rotation. It is a *vade mecum* meant to help them and other allied health professionals survive the neurology rotation through the provision of insightful guidelines and relevant images rather than to serve as an oversized reference text. An attempt has been made to keep the structure of every topic similar so as to aid students as they develop their thinking process in a stepwise fashion. A very brief introduction of each case has been provided as well.

This book is primarily intended for medical students; however, general medical residents, allied health professionals, nurse practitioners, physician assistants and other primary medical care providers who need a readily available and easily portable neuroradiology atlas and source book as they navigate through neurology rotations, training and ultimately their own practice, may find this book useful as well.

We do not present an exhaustive list of every possible neuroimaging condition, but provide a rational approach to imaging interpretation, including some fundamental physics of the basis of the different modalities. All of the information presented in this manual has been carefully reviewed for accuracy of the information presented to describe generally accepted practices. However the authors, editor and publisher are not responsible for the errors, omissions or consequences from the application of this information and make no expressed or implied warranty of the contents of this publication. The authors have made every effort to ensure that the explanations set forth in this text are in accordance with current recommendations and practice at the time of publication. In view of ongoing research and the constant flow of information, the reader is urged to check for regular updates as they become available. Suggestions to improve this publication are welcome and should be directed to the authors.

We are very grateful to our colleagues who archived the images of our mutual patients and retrieved them at request for this project: Dr. Myles Koby, neuroradiologist, Doctor's Community Hospital, Lanham, Maryland; Drs. Hee Lee and Gurmeet Sidhu, neuroradiologists at Prince George's Hospital Center, Cheverly, Maryland. We are also very thankful to our students Omar Syed (Canada), Ahmad Khan (Canada), Ifeoma Okadipo (USA) and intern Dr. Dejene Kasaye (USA), all of whom have worked tirelessly to retrieve the images and assist in the timely completion of this work. Thanks also to Paul Blankenship, RVT (USA), for archiving the ultrasound images of our ward patients.

Toronto, ON, Canada   Abdul Qayyum Rana
Cheverly, MD, USA   Lawrence A. Zumo
Edmonton, AB, Canada   Valerie Sim

Contents

x   Contents

Index to Cases

Chapter 1
Introductory Biochemical and Biophysical Principles

Abstract Neurology is a medical discipline which demands thorough history taking and precise localization based on physical examination. Neuroimaging modalities further aid the physician in diagnosing and managing of patients. In support of the dictum "insight before application", ascribed to Max Planck, we present a brief but critical summary of applicable biochemical and biophysical principles of neuroimaging and neurosonology. Major technologic advances in neuroradiology have resulted in the detection and better characterization of neurologic diseases; computerized tomography revolutionized clinical medicine in the 1970s, and magnetic resonance imaging has subsequently had a tremendous impact on neurologic practice. Fundamental principles of the most commonly encountered neuroimaging techniques are explained in this chapter, including CT, MRI, angiography, ultrasound, PET and SPECT.

1.1 Computerized Tomography (CT)

This modality utilizes cross sectional imagery based on the absorption of X-rays by biological tissues. Signal is measured in Hounsefield units (approximately −1,000 (air) to +1,000 (blood)), an arbitrary scale reflecting the attenuation coefficient of the differential attenuation properties of biological tissues. In modern machines, slice images are acquired at discrete intervals,

A.Q. Rana et al., *Neuroradiology in Clinical Practice*,
DOI 10.1007/978-3-319-01002-1_1,
© Springer International Publishing Switzerland 2013

either in axial or coronal plane, and are then reformatted in any desired plane (2–5 mm average slice thickness) or as volumetric (3D) representation of the structures. In 1989, an improvement of CT scanning was introduced; spiral CT (helical or volume acquisition) allows data to be acquired continuously by constant rotation of the X-ray tube detector coupled with constant moving of patient on the gantry. This makes shorter scanning times possible and lowers the amount of contrast material required.

A CT scan is often the initial imaging modality used in neurological conditions. A complete CT scan can be done in 5 minutes or less. Acute haemorrhage is readily identified on CT. The main disadvantage of a CT scan is that the posterior fossa and brainstem are not as well visualized.

1.1.1   CT Densities and Windowing

For CT images, signal is referred to as density. Whiter areas are hyperdense, darker areas are hypodense. A CT scan is a better tool for imaging bone structures, acute hemorrhage, and calcification, all of which appear hyperdense (white). Cerebrospinal fluid (CSF) is hypodense compared to brain, and air appears black. Different "window" settings can be selected, allowing details to be seen within the bone (bone windows) or the brain (brain window) (Fig. 1.1).

1.1.2   CT Contrast

CT scans can be obtained with and without intravenous contrast. Iodine-based dyes are the most common dyes used. Contrast dye can leach through a disrupted blood–brain barrier, as seen with tumours or inflammatory lesions, leaving behind contrast which is radio-opaque, and thus visible by CT. The major side effect of concern, apart from allergic reaction, is nephrotoxicity which probably occurs in less than 1 % of normal individuals, but can be as high as 10–20 % of people with chronic kidney disease. Renal function should always be assessed before administering contrast.

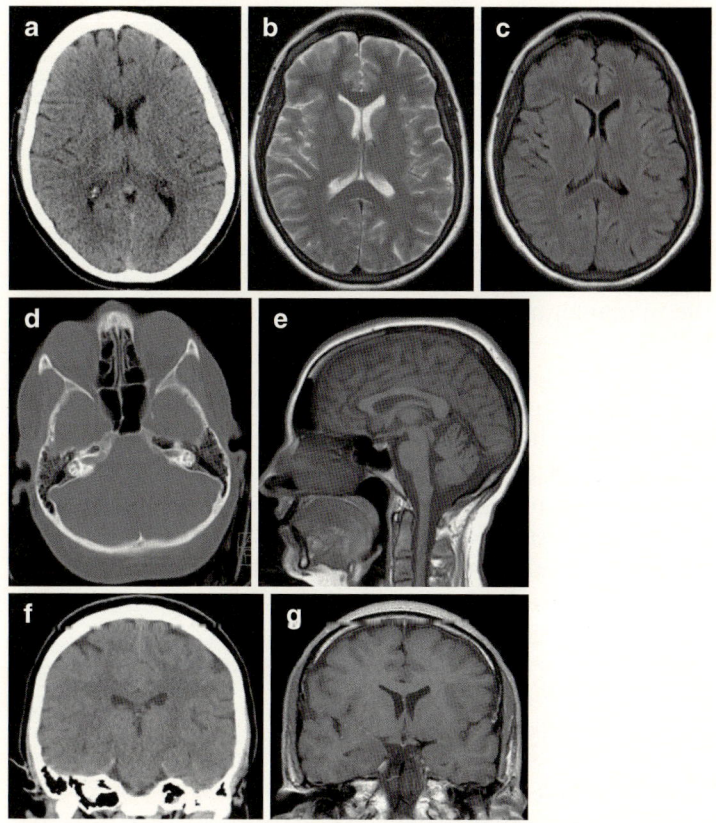

FIGURE 1.1 Imaging planes and CT/T1/T2/FLAIR examples. (a) Axial CT; (b) Axial T2-weighted MRI; (c) Axial FLAIR MRI; (d) Axial CT bone window; (e) Sagittal T1 MRI; (f) Coronal CT; (g) Coronal T1 MRI

1.1.3   CT Angiography (CTA)

Blood vessels can also be imaged using contrast dye. The bone densities are subtracted from the final image, leaving high resolution images of the intraluminal flow of neck and intracranial vessels (see Fig. 11.4).

1.2   Magnetic Resonance Imaging (MRI)

An MRI scan will take 20 minutes or much longer, depending on the sequences used, but provides more detailed information than CT scan about inflammatory lesions and posterior fossa or brainstem pathology. There are many different types of MRI sequences and these can seem confusing at first glance. To more easily identify and interpret the MRI scan types, it is important to understand some of the fundamentals of MRI physics. A simplified explanation follows.

MRI is based on nuclear magnetic resonance (NMR), a technique originally used by scientists for chemical analysis of molecules. It relies on calculations and extrapolations of magnetic relaxation times of nuclear particles. For clinical MRI, hydrogen protons are the particles analyzed, as these protons have significant magnetic moments (existing in the nucleus without associated neutrons) and are extremely abundant in tissues.

1.2.1   Spins and Magnetic Fields

Protons are positively charged particles at the centre of all atomic nuclei. Because they are always spinning and are charged, they create small magnetic fields, like tiny bar magnets. Thus protons have both a spin and a magnetic dipole. We humans are full of protons, but the spins and dipoles are random so all net dipole is zero (ie. we are not magnetized). However, when we are put into an MRI magnet, some of the dipoles align themselves with the magnetic field (in essence magnetizing the tissue to a small degree, enough to interfere with pacemakers, which is why this is an important screening question before any person enters the magnet!). More dipoles line up in the direction of the field such that the sum of all dipole vectors is $0°$. This is the new baseline state.

1.2.2   Generating MRI Signals

Once tissue is in this baseline magnetized state with the net dipole pointing to 0°, a radiofrequency pulse can be given. This causes the protons to enter a higher energy state, flipping to orient at 180°. As more protons "flip", the net dipole vector increases, becoming 90° when there are equal protons in both states. In the MRI machine, a receiver is located at 90° to the baseline state; the magnetic field at 90° induces a current (signal) in this receiver, proportional to the field strength. As soon as the radiofrequency pulse is stopped, the signal in this receiver "decays" as protons flip back to their baseline state. This decay, or relaxation, has two main forms for the purposes of clinical neuroradiology, T1 and T2 (measured in milliseconds):

T1-longitudinal (spin lattice) relaxation time: This is the time it takes for the net dipole to completely return to 0° from 90° after the radiofrequency pulse is stopped; that is, the time when the 90° receiver no longer has current induced by magnetic field from the tissue. It is strongly dependent on MRI field strength. Larger fields give better anatomic resolution in T1-weighted images. Most clinical MRIs use magnets of at least 3 T (60,000 times the earth's magnetic field).

T2-transverse nuclear spin magnetization decoherence: When protons spin, they act like a top which is about to fall over, that is, they wobble around a central axis. This movement is called precession. The precession of protons is random (incoherent) at baseline, even after being put into the MRI machine. Once a radiofrequency pulse is given, it causes excited protons to precess in synchronization (coherently). This precessional frequency can then be detected by the 90° receiver once the radiofrequency pulse is stopped. The T2 relaxation time is the time it takes for the synchronization of precession to disappear or become incoherent again. T2 is less dependent on magnetic field so larger MRI fields have less effect on T2 image quality.

TABLE 1.1 Intensity (MRI) and density (CT) characteristics of different substances

General	T1	T2	CT
Grey matter	Low	High	High
White matter	High	Low	Low
Calcium (bone cortex)	Low	Low	High
Fat (bone marrow)	High	Iso/low	Low
Edema, demyelination, infarction	Low	High	Iso/low
CSF	Low	High[a]	Low
Air	Low	Low	Low
Blood			
Hyperacute (intracellular oxyhemoglobin)	Iso/low	High/iso	High
1–2 days, acute (intracellular deoxyhemoglobin)	Iso	Low	High
2–7 days, early subacute (intracellular methemoglobin)	High	Low	Iso
1–4 weeks, late subacute (extracellular methemoglobin)	High	High	Iso/low
>2–6 weeks, chronic (intracellular hemosiderin)	Low	Low	Low

[a]On standard T2-weighted images, CSF is hyperintense; however, on FLAIR images, which are also T2-weighted, CSF is hypointense. Therefore, an image with low CSF signal can be T1 or T2-weighted (FLAIR); an image with high CSF signal must be a T2-weighted image

1.2.3   T1 and T2 Intensities (Table 1.1)

For MRI images, signal is referred to as intensity. Whiter areas are hyperintense, darker areas are hypointense. A short relaxation time produces a high signal (hyperintense); long relaxation gives low signal (hypointense).

<u>T1-weighted images</u>: ideal for displaying anatomical structures; less sensitive to water. Grey matter is hypointense (greyer), white matter hyperintense (whiter).

<u>T2-weighted images</u>: ideal for displaying pathology; more sensitive to water. Grey matter appears hyperintense (whiter), white matter hypointense (greyer).

1.2.4   Other MRI Sequences

By administering additional radiofrequency pulses during the decay processes, the signal from select protons can be cancelled out. For example, by timing when the pulses are given, signal from fat or water can be removed from the final image.

<u>Fluid attenuated inversion recovery (FLAIR)</u>: T2-weighted images in which the signal from CSF is cancelled out. Thus the CSF appears black. This should not be confused with a T1-weighted image, in which the CSF is also black. Removing CSF signal allows brain parenchyma lesions to be more visible (eg. periventricular hyperintense demyelination plaques of multiple sclerosis).

<u>Diffusion weighted imaging (DWI) and apparent diffusion coefficient (ADC)</u>: measures the diffusion of water protons and is used commonly in acute stroke, tumours and Creutzfeldt-Jakob disease. "Restricted diffusion" is thought to represent cytotoxic edema in the setting of acute stroke. The ADC should always be examined when interpreting diffusion weighted signals. True restricted diffusion will appear hypointense on ADC and hyperintense on DWI. Hyperintensity on DWI without corresponding hypointensity on ADC may reflect T2 shine-through only, not restricted diffusion.

<u>Fat suppression</u>: suppresses the normal hyperintense signal of fat, allowing better visualization of structures or lesions within areas of high fat (eg. orbits).

<u>Gradient recalled echo (GRE)</u>: sensitive to small amounts of blood, eg. within hemangiomas or other vascular malformations which may have bled in the past.

Magnetic transfer contrast: T1 weighted images which decrease white matter signal, allowing post-contrast T1 enhancing lesions to be better visualized.

Proton density: midway between a T1 and T2 image. It is also used to distinguish periventricular pathology, such as white matter demyelination, from CSF. Flow voids appear hypointense on both T1 and T2 images. They signify high-speed blood flow, as observed in arteriovenous malformations

Perfusion pulse sequence: better quantifies regional blood flow since it combines fast imaging techniques with IV contrast administration leading to better difference reflection of cerebral blood volume over time.

Echo planar imaging: ideal for uncooperative patients since it allows the rapid collection of imaging data in a very short time, approximately 50–100 ms.

1.2.5   MRI Contrast

Unlike CT contrast agents that are directly visualized, these are paramagnetic contrast agents (eg. gadolinium) that produce local alterations in the magnetic environment. This influences the MRI signal intensity which in turn influences the proton relaxation times. This signal change is what is visualized, not the contrast agent itself. These dyes are considered less nephrotoxic than CT dyes, but cases of nephrogenic systemic fibrosis are reported.

1.2.6   MR Angiography (MRA)

Time of flight angiography or phase contrast angiography are the two types of MRA used. Only the latter requires contrast. Intracranial and neck vessels can be imaged (see Figs. 11.2 and 11.3).

1.2.7   MR Venography (MRV)

MRV visualizes the venous system in the head and neck in order to identify certain pathologies such as dural sinus thrombosis. Gadolinium is injected and the VESPA (venous enhanced subtracted peak) approach is used to generate the image.

1.2.8   Functional MRI (fMRI)

Functional MRI measures brain activity by detecting changes in blood flow when a certain area of the brain is more active. It takes advantage of the blood oxygenation level dependent (BOLD) effect. In activated areas of the brain, venous blood is more oxygenated because of increased local blood flow with little change in oxygen consumption.

1.2.9   MR Spectroscopy (MRS)

MRS allows for the analysis of the chemical composition of certain areas of the brain and can help distinguish some neoplasms, infections and strokes. The main signals are from N-acetylaspartate (NAA), choline and lactate. NAA is a byproduct of the neurotransmitter glutamate and so is localized primarily to synaptic terminals. Decreases in NAA suggest neuronal loss. Choline is found in cell membranes and is generally increased in tumours and decreased in strokes. Lactate indicates anaerobic metabolism, as seen in necrotic tumours, infections or strokes.

1.3   Positron Emission Tomography (PET) and Single Photon Emission Tomography (SPECT)

Both PET and SPECT use ionizing radiation. Radioactivity of PET is in absolute units hence can be calibrated, but it is more expensive than SPECT. SPECT is less sensitive but is not plagued by motion problems as in PET. Each has their operational advantages.

The PET scan measures metabolism using 18-fluorodeoxyglucose uptake. The SPECT scan measures perfusion using isotopes in the blood. PET or SPECT signals can be increased in tumours. In seizures, signals are increased during active seizure and decreased at the seizure focus in between seizures. Signal patterns may help distinguish types of dementia also, with frontotemporal signal loss in frontotemporal dementias, and signal loss in the hippocampus, mesial parietal lobe and lateral parietotemporal cortex in Alzheimer's disease. In addition, a new amyloid tracer (11C-labelled Pittsburgh compound B) can be used in PET scans to identify amyloid lesions as seen in Alzheimer's disease.

1.4   Ultrasonography

"Ultrasono" implies sound wave frequencies higher than human hearing (more than 20,000 Hz). It is a safe imaging technique with no radiation exposure. Ultrasonographic machines use probes containing piezoelectric crystals that change shape when a current is applied to them. Rapid current oscillations produce rapid piezo expansions and contractions that are converted into acoustic energy (sound waves). The sound waves travel from the probe through biological tissues until they hit structures that reflect the waves back towards the probe. These "echo" waves are then recaptured and analyzed. Most ultrasound probes have frequency ranges of 2–10 MHz. In neurology, ultrasound it is used primarily to image blood vessels in the setting of stroke.

1.4.1   Doppler Ultrasonography

The Doppler effect, the key principle of vascular ultrasonography, is based on the change or shift in frequency (or wavelength) of a sound wave caused by relative movement between the sound source (scatterer) and the receiver. The Doppler frequency shift is the difference between the reflected frequency and the transmitted frequency. Blood flowing towards the probe produces positive Doppler frequency shifts, whilst that flowing away from the probe produces negative shifts.

The Doppler frequency shift (Fs) depends on the speed of the blood flow, the angle between the direction of sound beam and the direction of blood flow (insonation angle, theta), the transmitted frequency (F{t}) and the speed of sound in biological soft tissue (C). Since the frequency of the probe, the angle of insonation (60° or less for carotid, 0° for transcranial) and speed of sound in soft biological tissues (1,540 m/s) are known, the velocity of the sound source can be calculated.

Equation for calculation of velocity:

$$V(cm/s) = \frac{Fs(kHz) \times 77}{F(t)(MHz) \times \cos(theta)}$$

1.4.2 Carotid Doppler

There are three recognized methods of calculating stenosis angiographically (ECST method, NASCET method and the CC method). However, because of variance in the standardized methods for velocity/stenosis correlations, the NASCET (North American Carotid Stenosis Trial) method is the more recognized and used (Fig. 1.2).

Consensus parameters for grading carotid stenosis are based on peak systolic velocity (PSV) from the internal carotid artery (ICA), plaque estimate and the ratio of PSV from ICA to the common carotid artery (CCA) (Grant et al. 2003). They are shown in Table 1.2.

1.4.3 Transcranial Doppler (TCD)

This technique takes advantage of areas of less or no bone through which the ultrasound probe can detect blood vessels of the intracranial cerebral arteries. It is quite technician-dependent but can non-invasively identify intracranial stenoses.

FIGURE 1.2 Methods of calculating carotid stenosis. NASCET used the formula 1 – (a/c) where a is the residual lumen diameter at the maximum stenosis and c is the lumen diameter at a disease-free point above the stenosis. ECST used the formula 1 – (a/b) where b is the estimated lumen diameter at the level of the stenosis based on a visual impression of where the normal wall was before stenosis occurred. *ICA* internal carotid artery, *ECA* external carotid artery, *CCA* common carotid artery (Ferguson et al. 1999)

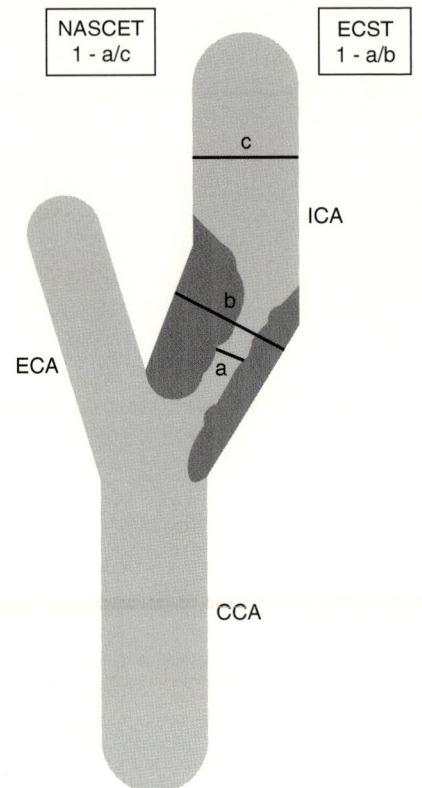

TABLE 1.2 Consensus parameters for grading carotid artery stenosis

Degree of stenosis	ICA PSV (cm/s)	Plaque estimate	ICA/CCA PSV ratio
Normal	<125	None	<2.0
<50 %	<125	<50	<2.0
50–69 %	125–230	≥50	2.0–4.0
≥70 %, less than near occlusion	>230	≥50	>4.0
Near occlusion	High, low, or undetectable	Visible	Variable
Total occlusion	Undetectable	Visible, no lumen	N/A

Adapted from Grant et al. (2003)

It can also actively monitor vasospasm, ongoing emboli, or recanalization post-tPA in acute stroke.

1.5 Angiography

A cerebral angiography presents high-quality images of the intracranial and extracranial cerebral blood vessels. This test involves inserting a catheter into the femoral artery and manipulating the tip into the cerebral vessels where radio-opaque dye is directly injected while Xray images are taken. Angiography is the gold standard for diagnosing certain conditions, including vasculitis, arteriovenous malformations and aneurysms.

Angiography carries a 1–2 % risk of stroke during the procedure as well as allergic reactions to the dye, nephrotoxicity from the dye, infections at the site of catheter introduction, excessive bleeding, blood clots, femoral nerve injury and even death.

References

Ferguson GG, Eliasziw M, Barr HW, et al. The North Amercian Symptomatic Carotid Endarterectomy Trial: surgical results in 1415 patients. Stroke. 1999;30(9):1751–8.

Grant EG, Benson CB, Moneta GL, et al. Carotid artery stenosis: gray-scale and Doppler US diagnosis – Society of Radiologists in Ultrasound Consensus Conference. Radiology. 2003;229(2):340–6.

Chapter 2
Vascular Disorders

Abstract In acute stroke, CT is the first modality of choice. A hyperacute ischemic stroke may appear normal or as blurring of the gray-white junction. At this stage, there is no enhancement with contrast. Acute ischemic stroke appears as an ill-defined hypodensity. There is usually no enhancement or only slight gyral enhancement at this stage. Subacute ischemic stroke appears a clear hypodensity with gyral enhancement. Acute and subacute haemorrhages appear hyperdense, whereas remote hemorrhages are hypodense. MRI diffusion weighting is helpful in demonstrating the restricted diffusion (cytotoxicity) of acute stroke and detecting smaller posterior fossa and brainstem infarcts. In this chapter, cases of ischemic and haemorrhagic stroke are presented.

A.Q. Rana et al., *Neuroradiology in Clinical Practice*,
DOI 10.1007/978-3-319-01002-1_2,
© Springer International Publishing Switzerland 2013

Case 2.1 Stroke Evolution
A 66 year-old left-handed female with a history of previous right parietal stroke presented with a 1 h history of sudden onset right hemiplegia and aphasia. CT and MRI imaging at 1 and 24 h was performed (Fig. 2.1).

Explanation and Diagnosis
The CT scan at 1 h (Fig. 2.1a) shows a hypodense old right parietal infarct and also early ischemia in the left middle cerebral artery territory: loss of grey-white junction in the anterior parietal lobe and loss of definition of the internal capsule. The areas of damage are better demonstrated as hypodensities on the CT scan at 24 h (Fig. 2.1b). MRI diffusion weighted and ADC images (Fig. 2.1c, d) also reveal the extent of acute ischemia. Clinically this woman's deficit did not resolve.

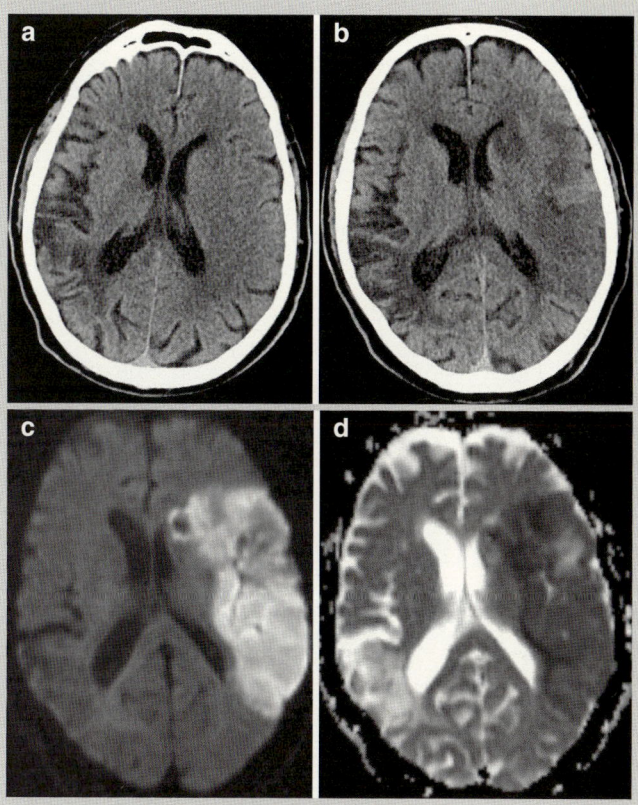

FIGURE 2.1 Axial imaging of left middle cerebral artery stroke in evolution. (**a**) CT at 1 h; (**b**) CT at 24 h; (**c**) Diffusion weighted (DWI) MRI; (**d**) Apparent diffusion coefficient (ADC) MRI

Case 2.2 Acute Stroke: Sulcal Effacement

A 57 year-old right-handed male presented with a sudden onset of right hemiplegia and aphasia. He was imaged within 12 h of onset (Fig. 2.2).

Explanation and Diagnosis

Figure 2.2 shows a left frontoparietal sulcal effacement as well as a loss of grey-white junction. Clinically this man's deficit did not resolve.

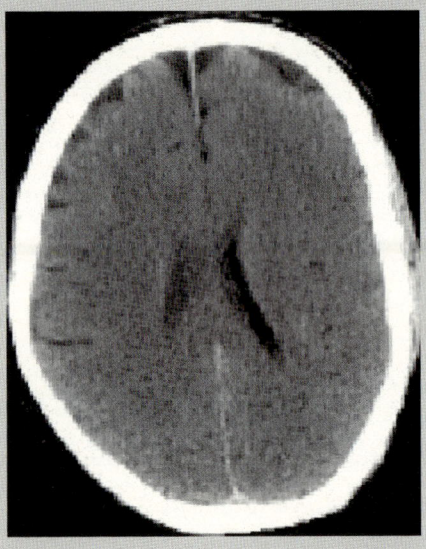

FIGURE 2.2 Axial CT scan of acute left middle cerebral artery stroke

Case 2.3 Haemorrhagic Transformation

A 63 year-old right-handed male presented with a sudden onset of expressive aphasia and right hemiparesis. A CT scan was done after 24 h (Fig. 2.3).

Explanation and Diagnosis

Figure 2.3 shows an area of hypodensity in the left fronto-parietal region consistent with subacute ischemic infarction in the middle cerebral artery territory. In addition, there is hyperdensity within the ischemic area consistent with haemorrhagic transformation. Clinically this patient's deficit was persistent.

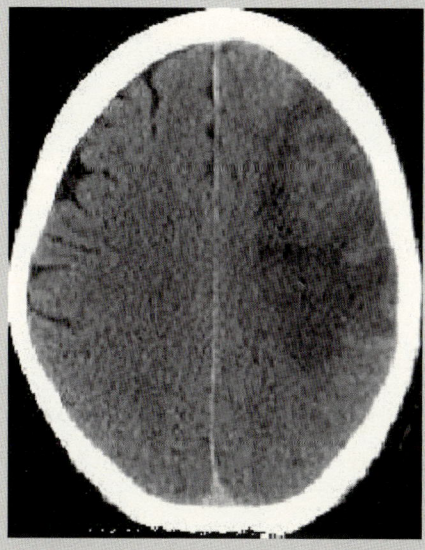

FIGURE 2.3 Axial CT scan showing subacute left middle cerebral artery stroke with haemorrhagic transformation

Case 2.4 Posterior Circulation Stroke

A 55 year-old right-handed female presented with a sudden onset right homonymous hemianopia, word finding problems and right hemiparesis. She later developed a left homonymous hemianopia. An MRI was performed (Fig. 2.4).

Explanation and Diagnosis

Figure 2.4 shows a large hyperintense signal abnormality involving left occipito-temporal area and a smaller hyperintensity of the right occipital lobe consistent with posterior circulation infarcts. Clinically this woman's deficits partially resolved.

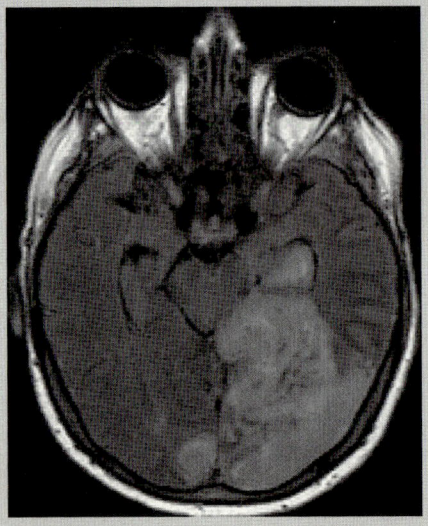

FIGURE 2.4 Axial FLAIR MRI showing bilateral posterior cerebral artery territory infarcts

Case 2.5 Thalamic Stroke

A 41 year-old right handed female presented with difficulty finding words during conversation and her speech was grammatically incorrect. The rest of the neurological examination was normal. An MRI was performed (Fig. 2.5).

Explanation and Diagnosis

Figure 2.5 shows a hyperintense lesion in left thalamus consistent with an acute thalamic ischemic infarct. Clinically this patient improved with speech therapy.

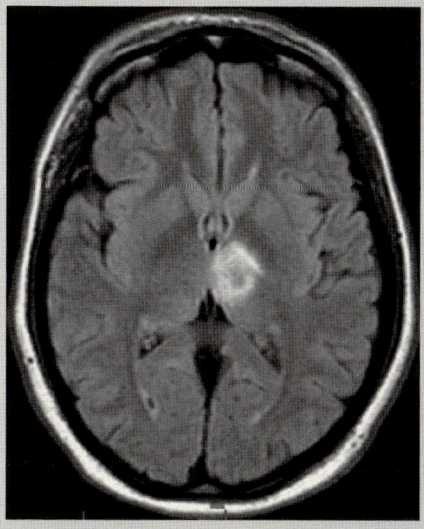

FIGURE 2.5 Axial FLAIR MRI showing left thalamic stroke

Case 2.6 Lacunar Stroke

A 65 year-old right handed male presented with a sudden onset of left arm weakness which started improving after 2–3 h. He presented 15 h after the onset, by which time his neurological examination only revealed a pronator drift of the left arm. A CT scan was done (Fig. 2.6).

Explanation and Diagnosis

Figure 2.6 shows a small right posterior frontal hypodensity consistent with ischemia of the primary motor cortex in the right middle cerebral artery branch distribution. Clinically this patient fully recovered.

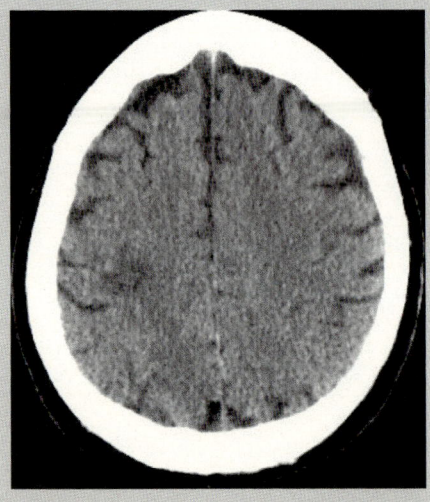

Figure 2.6 Axial CT showing right posterior frontal lacunar infarct

Case 2.7 Haemorrhagic Stroke

A 65 year-old female with a history of hypertension presented with a sudden onset of right sided weakness and numbness. She had stopped taking her anti-hypertensive medication a few weeks prior to the onset of symptoms. A CT scan without contrast was performed on presentation (Fig. 2.7).

Explanation and Diagnosis

Figure 2.7 shows a hyperdensity in the left basal ganglia and internal capsule region. The findings are consistent with an acute left intracerebral hemorrhage likely due to uncontrolled hypertension. Clinically the patient improved with rehabilitation.

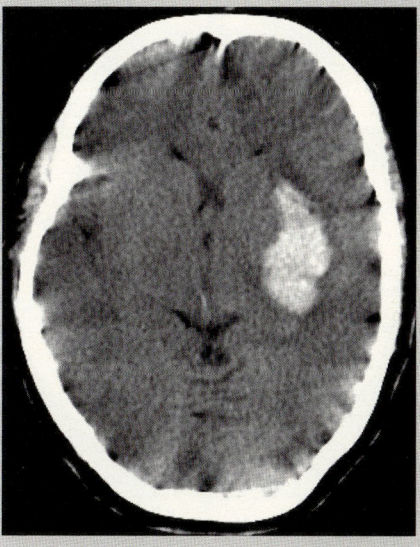

FIGURE 2.7 Axial CT showing haemorrhage in the left basal ganglia and internal capsule

Case 2.8 Subarachnoid Haemorrhage

A 42 year-old male presented with a sudden onset of acute severe headache and a decline in level of consciousness. There was significant neck stiffness on examination. A CT scan was performed urgently (Fig. 2.8).

Explanation and Diagnosis

Figure 2.8 shows hyperdensites in the basal cisterns and major fissures of the brain consistent with acute subarachnoid hemorrhage from a ruptured aneurysm. Clinically this patient developed hydrocephalus and did not survive.

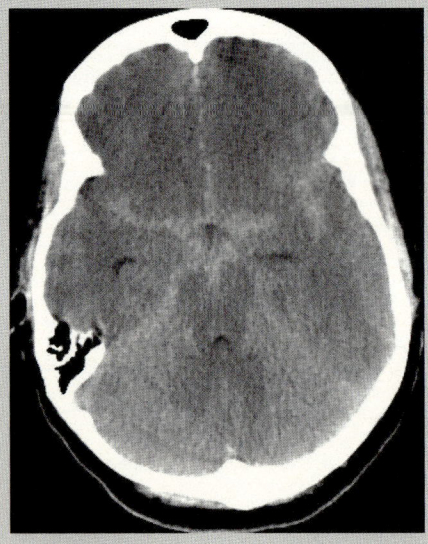

FIGURE 2.8 Axial CT showing subarachnoid haemorrhage in the basal cisterns

Case 2.9 Anoxic Brain Injury

A 50 year-old male was brought to the emergency room via ambulance after being found with an extended period of altered mental status of unknown etiology. A CT scan was performed (Fig. 2.9).

Explanation and Diagnosis

Figure 2.9 shows complete loss of grey-white differentiation and evidence of ischemia (hypodensity) to the caudate nuclei bilaterally. This is consistent with profound anoxic brain injury. Clinically this patient did not survive.

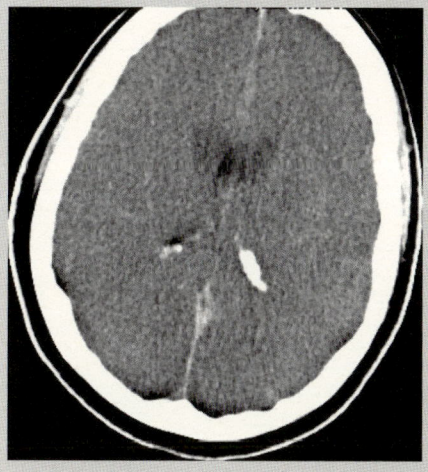

FIGURE 2.9 Axial CT showing diffuse cerebral edema and caudate ischemia

Chapter 3
White Matter Diseases and Demyelination

Abstract There are many diseases and syndromes which affect the white matter of the brain. The most common by far is multiple sclerosis, but the differential includes infectious, inflammatory, metabolic, mitochondrial, vascular, neoplastic and toxic etiologies. In this chapter we present the 2010 McDonald MRI diagnostic criteria for multiple sclerosis and include example cases of mulitple sclerosis, transverse myelitis, autoimmune encephalitis, toxic demyelination, posterior reversible encephalopathy syndrome and neuroBechet's disease. Progressive multifocal leukoencephalopathy is presented under infectious diseases (Chap. 9), CNS lymphoma is presented under Tumours (Chap. 4), and osmotic demyelination is presented under metabolic disorders (Chap. 10).

McDonald Criteria for Diagnosis of Multiple Sclerosis

For a patient to be diagnosed with multiple sclerosis, he or she must have evidence of demyelination which is disseminated in space and time. MRI can support the diagnosis, as defined the McDonald criteria, most recently revised in 2010 (Polman et al. 2011). Separation in space is met by one or more hyperintense lesions on T2-weighted imaging in at least two of four regions (periventricular, juxtacortical, infratentorial or spinal cord). Separation in time is met by the simultaneous presence of asymptomatic enhancing and non-enhancing lesions, or new T2 or enhancing lesions on subsequent MRI scans.

A.Q. Rana et al., *Neuroradiology in Clinical Practice*,
DOI 10.1007/978-3-319-01002-1_3,
© Springer International Publishing Switzerland 2013

Case 3.1 Multiple Sclerosis (FLAIR Sequences)
A 43 year old right-handed female presented with progressive numbness from her right axilla to her trunk to both legs. There was no problem with her vision, speech, or swallowing. She had no weakness, bowel or bladder symptoms. Her symptoms resolved over the next 4 weeks. Three months later she developed persistent numbness on the left side, which resolved after 3 weeks. An MRI was performed (Fig. 3.1).

Explanation and Diagnosis
Figure 3.1 shows multiple asymmetrical oval hyperintense signal abnormalities which are disseminated in space and are consistent with demyelination. Their ovoid appearance and projection from the corpus callosum (known as Dawson fingers) are typical for multiple sclerosis.

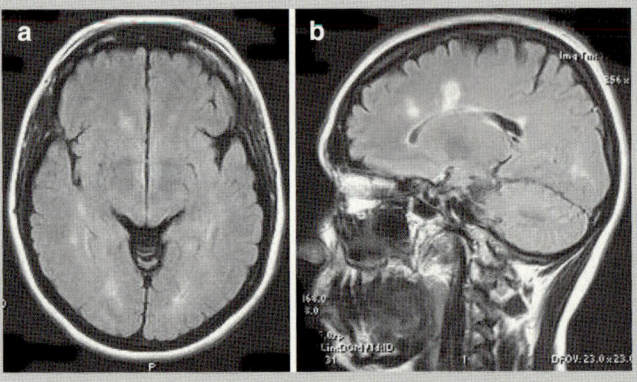

FIGURE 3.1 Axial (**a**) and sagittal (**b**) FLAIR MRI showing multiple areas of demyelination

Case 3.2 Multiple Sclerosis (T1 and T2 Sequences)

A 27 year old right-handed male presented with a gradual onset of blurred vision and numbness on the right side of his body which lasted for 3 weeks, after which the numbness resolved gradually. An MRI was performed (Fig. 3.2).

Explanation and Diagnosis

Figure 3.2a shows multiple white matter hyperintense signal abnormalities consistent with demyelination. Figure 3.2b shows multiple hypointense signal abnormalities involving the corpus callosum and subcortical white matter consistent with axonal loss. The combination of these findings are suggestive of multiple sclerosis.

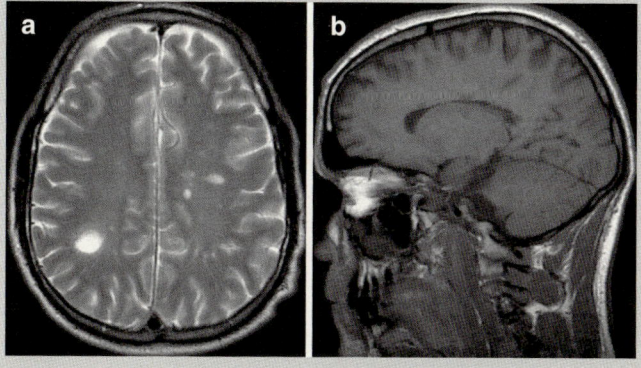

FIGURE 3.2 (a) Axial T2-weighted MRI showing multiple areas of demyelination; (b) sagittal T1-weighted MRI showing multiple hypointense signal abnormalities (black holes) involving the corpus callosum and subcortical white matter

Case 3.3 Transverse Myelitis

A 57 year old right-handed female presented with a tingling in her lower extremities. Upon neurological examination, she was found to have increased tone in the legs, hyperreflexia and extensor plantar responses. She also had a patchy sensory loss in both legs. An MRI scan of whole spine was performed (Fig. 3.3).

Explanation and Diagnosis

Figure 3.3 shows a hyperintense signal in the spinal cord at the C3-C5 level consistent with acute transverse myelitis. Transverse myelitis can occur with multiple sclerosis or other infectious/inflammatory conditions. Those associated with multiple sclerosis are generally associated with little or no cord swelling, span less than two vertebral segments, are clearly delineated and only involve a portion of the cord in cross section.

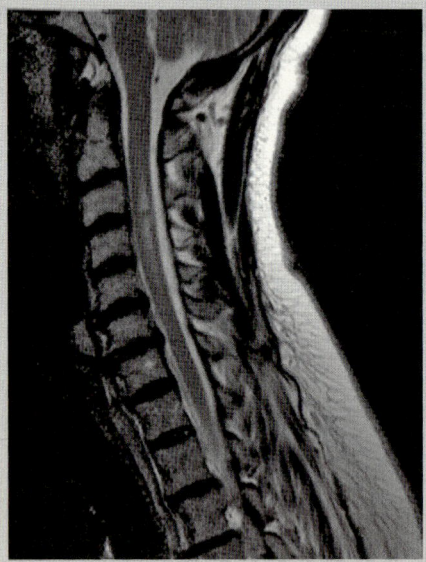

FIGURE 3.3 Sagittal T2-weighted MRI showing transverse myelitis

Case 3.4 Tumefactive Multiple Sclerosis

A 29 year old male (HIV negative, non-illicit drug abuser) presented to the emergency department with acute gait imbalance and 2 weeks of pain, progressive numbness and right hemiparesis.

Explanation and Diagnosis

Figure 3.4 shows a homogeneous T2 hyperintense lesion with surrounding vasogenic edema. The amount of edema is relatively small relative to the size of the lesion. The differential for such a lesion includes tumour, infection and demyelination. Without fever or other constitutional signs, abscess is less likely. Biopsy proved this lesion to be tumefactive multiple sclerosis.

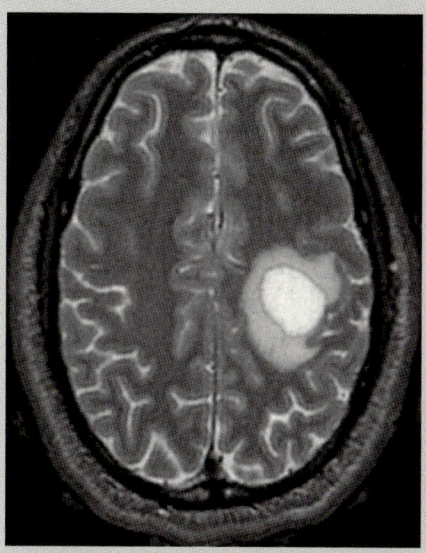

FIGURE 3.4 Left parietal lobe tumefactive demyelination

Case 3.5 Autoimmune Encephalitis

A 25 year old female presented with a subacute onset of confusion and headache and progressed to bilateral hemiparesis. Examination also revealed a left homonymous hemianopia. An MRI was performed (Fig. 3.5).

Explanation and Diagnosis

Figure 3.5 reveals extensive white matter and deep gray matter involvement as well as a stroke of the right occipital lobe. The U-fibres were spared, as often seen in leukodsytrophies. However, this patient had white cells in the cerebral spinal fluid. Infectious and vasculitic work-up was negative but she clinically resolved with steroid treatment leading to a presumed diagnosis of autoimmune encephalitis.

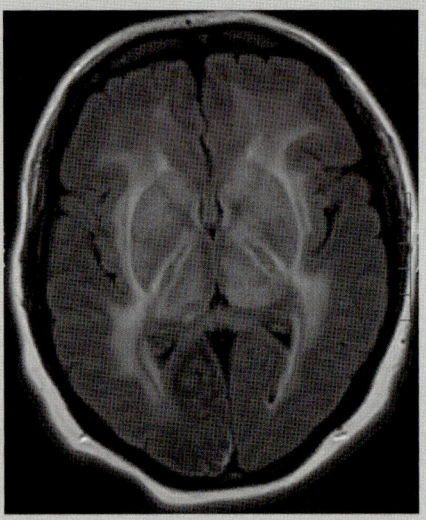

FIGURE 3.5 FLAIR MRI showing symmetrical hyperintensities of white matter and deep gray matter and ischemia of the right occipital lobe

Case 3.6 Toxic Demyelination (Levamisole Toxicity)

A 52 year old male with a remote history of cocaine use presented with a 3 months history of confusion, ataxia, dysarthria and a 30 lb weight loss. Work-up led to the diagnosis of squamous cell carcinoma of the lung. An MRI of the brain was also performed (Fig. 3.6).

Explanation and Diagnosis

The differential for ring-enhancing lesions as seen in Fig. 3.6 includes metastatic neoplasm, infection and inflammation. Given the concurrent diagnosis of lung cancer in this patient, these lesions were initially thought to be metastatic, but they do not show much edema and their location is more suggestive of demyelination. The lesions actually resolved with time and were concluded to be a toxic reaction to levamisole which had been cut into the cocaine this patient had previously used. After surgical resection of the lung cancer, this patient continues to do well.

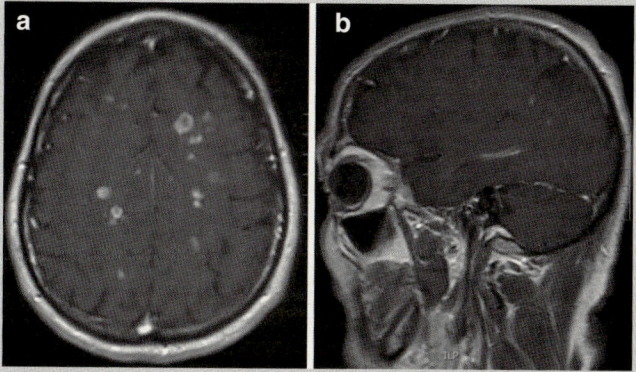

FIGURE 3.6 Axial (**a**) and sagittal (**b**) gadolinium-enhanced T1-weighted MRI showing multiple ring-enhancing demyelination lesions

Case 3.7 NeuroBeçhet's
A 23 year old right handed male awoke with right sided ataxic hemiparesis. He had a past history of migraines, joint pain, recurrent oral ulcers, an episode of genital ulcers, and a prior history of uveitis. A lumbar puncture showed 30 WBC, 66 % lymphs, 17 % mono, 16 % poly, 1 % eosin. Oligoclonal bands were negative and IgG levels were only slightly elevated. ESR was 20, but other bloodwork for inflammatory disease (ANA, ENA, ANCA, ACE, etc.) was normal. An MRI was performed (Fig. 3.7a)

Explanation and Diagnosis
Figure 3.7a shows T2 hyperintensity extending from the pons through left peduncle to internal capsule. Some diffusion change was present in part of the lesion, and there was some mild enhancement. The clinical picture and MRI findings are consistent with a diagnosis of neuroBeçhet's. Clinically he responded to high dose steroids. Two years later he developed symptoms on the other side. Repeat imaging (Fig. 3.7b) shows resolution of the prior lesion but development of a contralateral lesion.

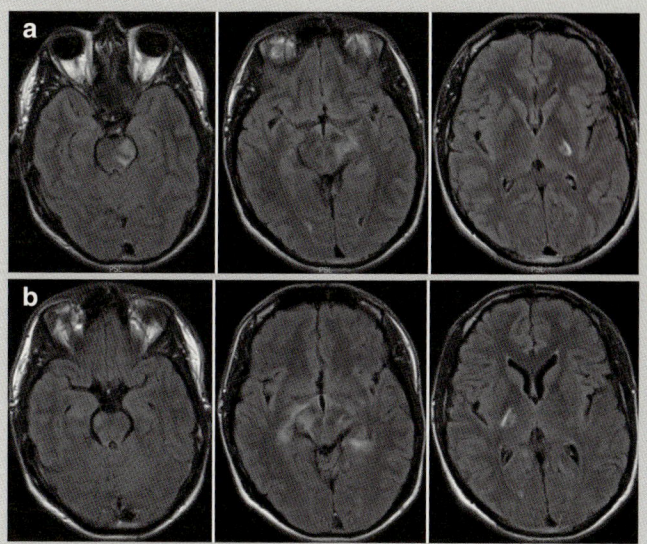

FIGURE 3.7 (**a**) Axial FLAIR MRIs showing hyperintense signal in the left pons through left peduncle and internal capsule consistent with NeuroBeçhet's. (**b**) Repeat imaging 2 years later showing resolution of old lesion and development of new lesion predominantly on the opposite side

Case 3.8 Posterior Reversible Encephalopathy Syndrome
A 19 year old female with no significant past medical history presented with shortness of breath, headache, hyperkalemia and acute renal failure, after 5 days of intense hiking under desert conditions without proper nutrition or hydration. Her BUN/Cr was 151/14.4 and her potassium was 7.3. She was intubated for airway protection and the hyperkalemia was corrected. She had two witnessed generalized seizures and developed cortical blindness. An MRI was performed (Fig. 3.8).

Explanation and Diagnosis
Figure 3.8 shows hyperintense signal in both occipital lobes consistent with vasogenic edema. There is no mass effect or hemorrhage. In this case, no restricted diffusion was seen (not shown), but diffusion changes can occur in this syndrome. The clinical picture and imaging is consistent with posterior reversible encephalopathy syndrome (PRES). Clinically, this patient recovered fully after hemodialysis.

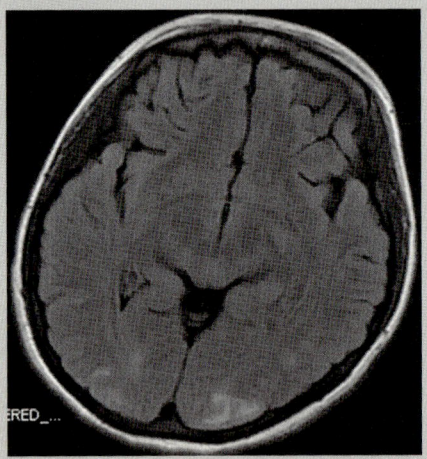

FIGURE 3.8 Axial FLAIR MRI showing bilateral occipital lobe vasogenic edema secondary to posterior reversible encephalopathy syndrome

Reference

Polman CH, Reingold SC, Banwell B, et al. Diagnostic criteria for multiple sclerosis: 2010 revisions to the McDonald criteria. Ann Neurol. 2011;69(2):292–302.

Chapter 4
Tumours

Abstract Tumours can occur anywhere in the nervous system and can be primary or metastatic. Many tumours can be identified based on their imaging characteristics. Tumours may be intra or extraaxial, hyper or hypointense, enhancing or nonenhancing, calcified or haemorrhagic. In this chapter we present some examples of primary and metastatic tumours, including glioblastoma multiforme, oligodendroglioma, meningiomas, schwannoma, solitary fibrous spinal tumour, lymphoma and metastatic lung cancer.

A.Q. Rana et al., *Neuroradiology in Clinical Practice*,
DOI 10.1007/978-3-319-01002-1_4,
© Springer International Publishing Switzerland 2013

Case 4.1 Glioblastoma Multiforme

A 65 year old male presented with a history of headaches causing early morning awakening, personality changes and a generalized seizure. An MRI was performed (Fig. 4.1).

Explanation and Diagnosis

Figure 4.1 shows a large mass in the left frontal lobe with edema and midline shift, as well as post-contrast ring enhancement. The findings are consistent with the primary brain tumor, glioblastoma multiforme (GBM).

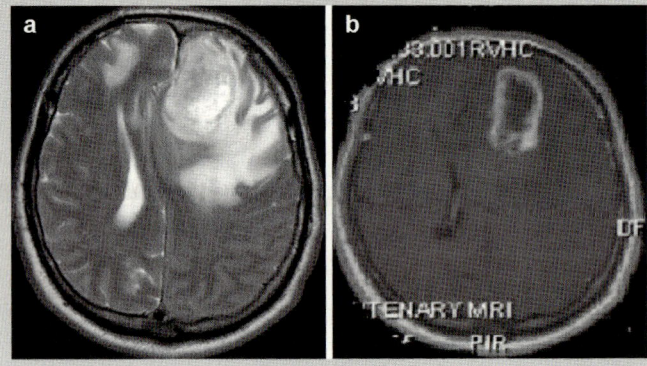

FIGURE 4.1 Axial T2-weighted (**a**) and post-contrast T1-weighted (**b**) MRI showing a left frontal lobe glioblastoma multiforme

Case 4.2 Oligodendroglioma

A 27 year old right-handed male presented with a gradual onset of headaches over several weeks, followed by multiple generalized seizures. A brain MRI was performed (Fig. 4.2).

Explanation and Diagnosis

Figure 4.2 shows a right occipital mass lesion consistent with oligodendroglioma.

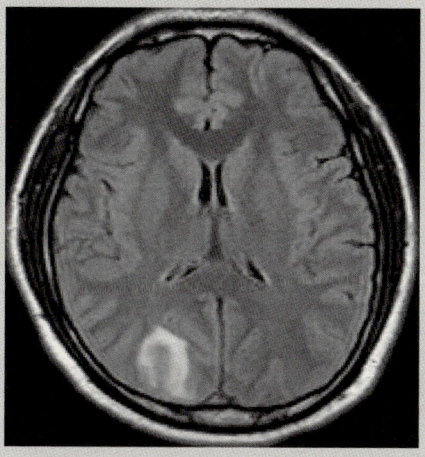

FIGURE 4.2 Axial FLAIR MRI image showing right occipital oligodendroglioma

Case 4.3 Meningioma

A 65 year old female presented with a history of falls when getting up to go to the bathroom in the middle of the night. She then had a generalized seizure lasting 2 min. An MRI was performed (Fig. 4.3).

Explanation and Diagnosis

Figure 4.3 shows a left frontal extra-axial lesion with diffuse enhancement, mass effect and vasogenic edema. A dural tail can also be seen. This was a left frontal meningioma.

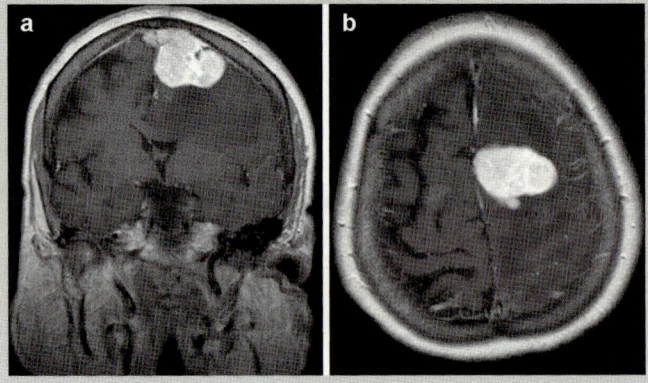

FIGURE 4.3 Coronal (**a**) and axial (**b**) enhanced T1-weighted MRI showing left frontal meningioma

Case 4.4 Interhemispheric Meningioma
A 58 year old right-handed female presented with two past episodes of a brief loss of consciousness accompanied with shaking of both sides of her body which lasted for about 2 min. There was no tongue biting or incontinence of the bowel or bladder. An MRI of brain was performed (Fig. 4.4).

Explanation and Diagnosis
Figure 4.4 shows a homogenously contrast enhancing extra-axial space occupying lesion attached to the mid line falx cerebri. The diagnosis was meningioma.

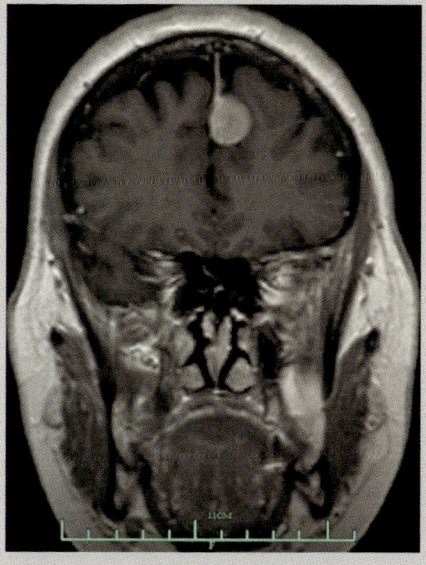

FIGURE 4.4 Coronal enhanced T1-weighted MRI showing an interhemispheric meningioma

Case 4.5 Schwannoma
A 38 year old right-handed male presented with an 8 month history of progressive left sided hearing loss and increased sensitivity to noise. Subsequently he developed constant left ear tinnitus. An MRI was performed (Fig. 4.5).

Explanation and Diagnosis
Figure 4.5 shows a homogenously enhancing mass lesion measuring 1.5 × 1.5 × 1.2 cm extending into the left internal auditory canal, consistent with left vestibular schwannoma (also known as acoustic neuroma).

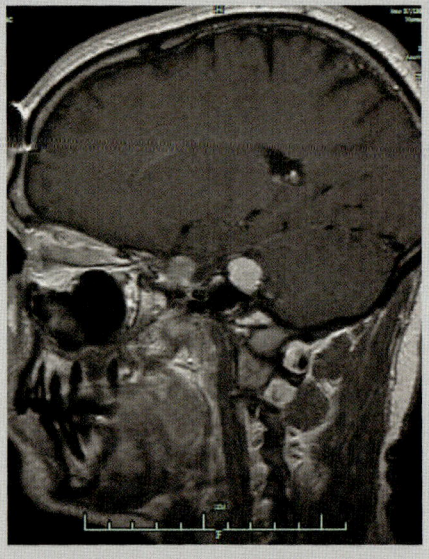

Figure 4.5 Sagittal enhanced T1-weighted MRI showing a left internal auditory canal Schwannoma

Case 4.6 Spinal Tumour

A 56 year old female presented with a 3 month history of gradual onset bilateral leg weakness. Upon examination she had mild weakness of both lower extremities with hyperreflexia and extensor plantar responses. She had a sensory level slightly above her umbilicus. An MRI scan of the spine was performed (Fig. 4.6).

Explanation and Diagnosis

Figure 4.6 shows a T2 hypointense focal mass lesion at T7. Most spinal tumours are hyperintense on T2 imaging, so the hypointensity in this case suggests the diagnosis of solitary fibrous tumour. T2 hypointensity can also occur with haemorrhage, as seen around ependymoma tumours, or with calcification. An extruded disc will also appear hypointense on T2.

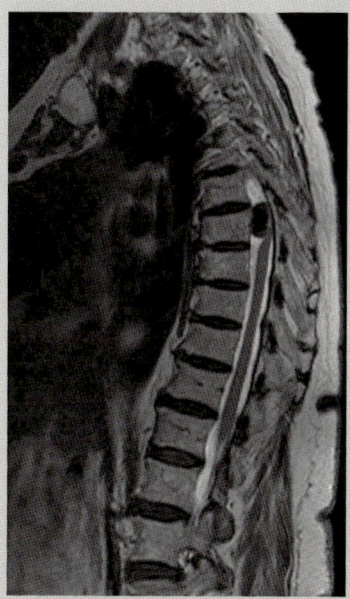

FIGURE 4.6 Sagittal T2-weighted MRI showing a hypointense fibrous tumour at T7 (Courtesy of I.U. Haq)

Case 4.7 CNS Lymphoma

A 40 year old female presented with headache, general malaise and loss of concentration. Pre and post-contrast CT and MRI scans were performed (Fig. 4.7).

Explanation and Diagnosis

Figure 4.7 shows a homogeneously enhancing lesion with surrounding vasogenic edema. Edema is seen as hypodense on CT (Fig. 4.7a) and hyperintense on T2-weighted MRI (Fig. 4.7b). This was proven by biopsy to be a B-cell lymphoma.

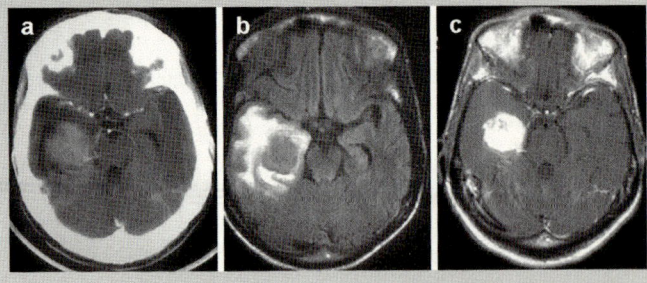

FIGURE 4.7 Right temporal lobe lymphoma. (a) Axial enhanced CT; (b) Axial FLAIR MRI; (c) Axial enhanced T1-weighted MRI

Case 4.8 Vertebral Metastasis

An 84 year-old female presented with weakness of both legs and difficulty walking. Upon neurological examination she was found to have decreased sensation up both legs. MRI scan of whole spine was performed (Fig. 4.8).

Explanation and Diagnosis

Figure 4.8 shows a metastatic lesion involving the T7 vertebral body with significant spinal cord compression and signal change. There is also mild cervical stenosis at C5-C6. Clinically this patient slowly became paraplegic and incontinent with loss of sensation up to xiphisternum.

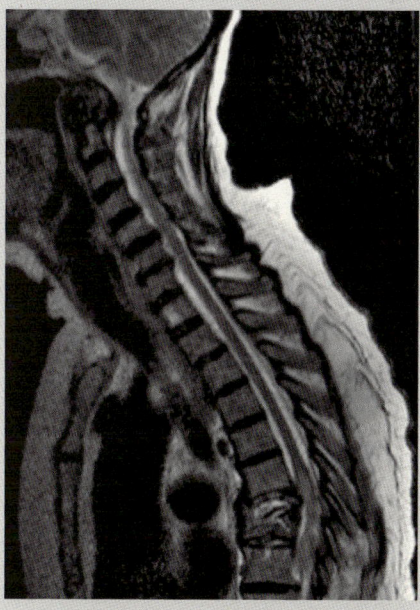

FIGURE 4.8 Sagittal T2-weighted MRI image showing a metastatic lesion involving T7 vertebral body

Case 4.9 Cerebral Metastasis

A 54 year old male with a 5 year history of recurrent non small cell lung carcinoma presented with headaches without fever, chills or rigors. CT and MRI scans were performed (Fig. 4.9).

Explanation and Diagnosis

Figure 4.9 shows ring enhancing lesions and surrounding vasogenic edema within the left parietal lobe. Only the hypodense edema can be clearly seen on CT (Fig. 4.9a). The MRI reveals T2 hyperintense edema and hypointense mass which ring-enhances (Fig. 4.9b, c). After steroid treatment, the amount of vasogenic edema is reduced (Fig. 4.9d). The diagnosis is metastatic non small cell lung carcinoma.

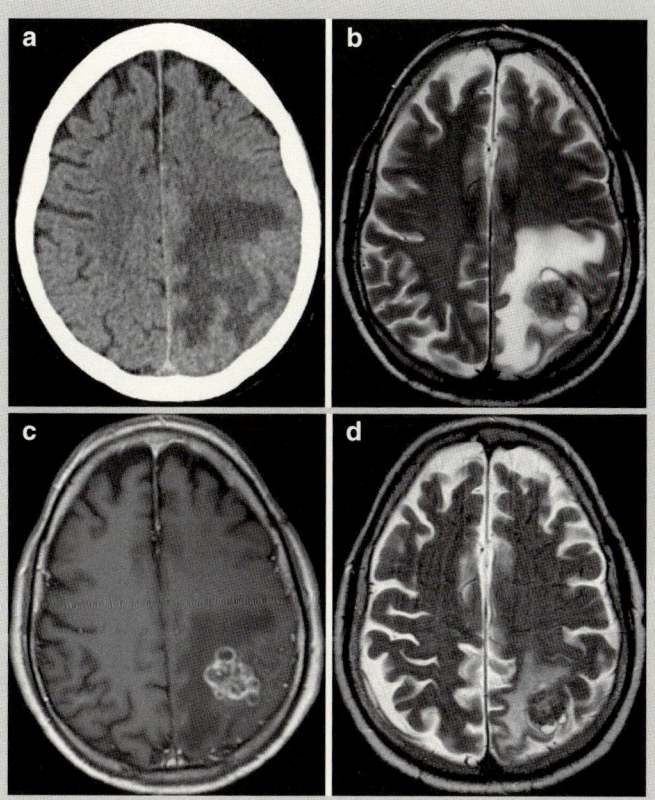

FIGURE 4.9 Axial images of left parietal lobe metastasis from non small cell lung cancer. (**a**) Non-contrast CT; (**b**) T2-weighted MRI; (**c**) Post-contrast T1-weighted MRI; (**d**) T2-weighted MRI after steroid treatment (Courtesy of M. Koby)

Chapter 5
Neurodegenerative Conditions

Abstract A number of degenerative conditions can affect the central nervous system and imaging modalities can be helpful in determining the diagnosis. Here we present cases of frontotemporal dementia, olivopontocerebellar atrophy, spinocerebellar ataxia, multiple systems atrophy, corticobasal degeneration, spinal muscular atrophy and Creutzfeldt-Jakob disease (CJD). CJD is sometimes classified under infectious diseases as it is transmissible, however it is truly a protein folding disease with more similarity to Alzheimer's and Parkinson's diseases than any infectious disease, so it is presented here instead.

Case 5.1 Frontotemporal Dementia
An 86 year old male presented with 2 years of gradual onset change in behaviour, lack of interest in activities and memory loss. On examination, frontal release signs were present and he was easily distracted. A CT scan of the brain was performed (Fig. 5.1).

Explanation and Diagnosis
Figure 5.1 shows prominent atrophy of frontal and temporal lobes with relative preservation of the occipital lobes. There is also some remote ischemic change of the left more than right subcortical frontal lobes, consistent with small vessel ischemic damage. This patient has frontotemporal dementia.

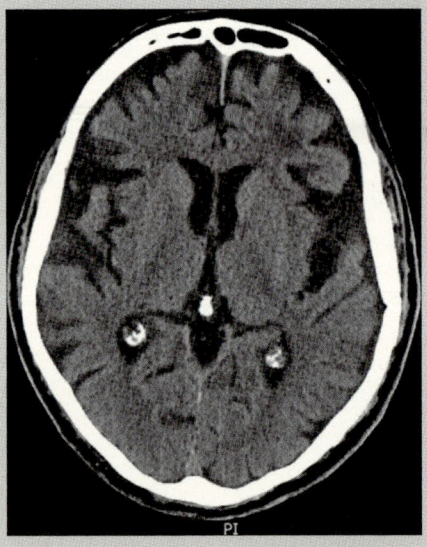

FIGURE 5.1 Axial CT showing significant bilateral frontal and temporal lobe atrophy and remote left frontal lobe subcortical ischemia

Case 5.2 Olivopontocerebellar Atrophy

A 37 year old right-handed female presented with speech problems and mild cognitive difficulties, as well as balance problems. Upon physical examination, she had mild dysarthria with scanning speech, finger-nose-finger and heel-knee-shin dysmetria. An MRI of the brain was performed (Fig. 5.2).

Explanation and Diagnosis

Figure 5.2 shows striking loss of cerebellar and pontine volume, consistent with a diagnosis of olivopontocerebellar atrophy.

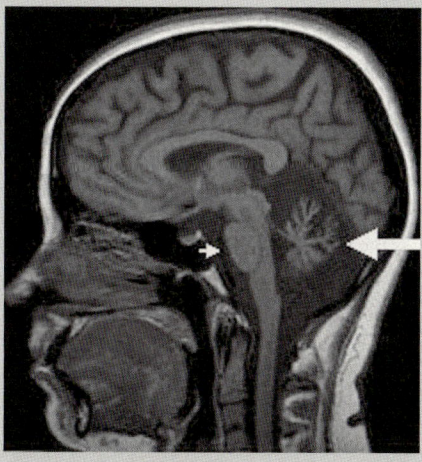

FIGURE 5.2 Sagittal T1-weighted MRI showing marked pontine (*short arrow*) and cerebellar (*large arrow*) atrophy

Case 5.3 Spinocerebellar Ataxia 3
A 42 year old right-handed female presented with a gradual onset of speech impairment and balance problems. Upon examination, she had spastic dysarthria, spasticity of upper and lower extremities, hyperreflexia, as well as a wide-based gait. An MRI was performed (Fig. 5.3).

Explanation and Diagnosis
Figure 5.3 shows mild generalized atrophy and severe cerebellar atrophy. The patient was diagnosed with Machado-Joseph Disease (Spinocerebellar ataxia type 3) through genetic testing.

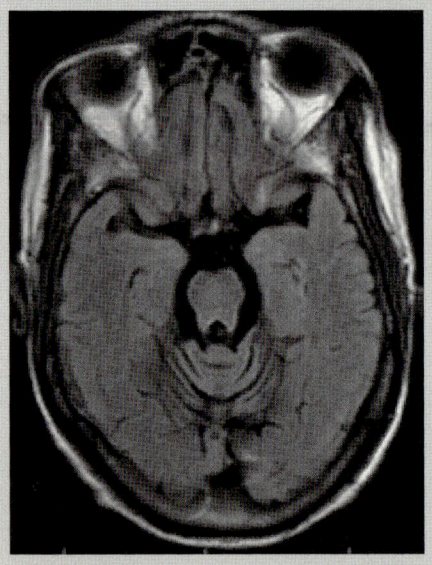

FIGURE 5.3 Axial FLAIR MRI showing pontine and cerebellar atrophy

Case 5.4 Spinocerebellar Ataxia 2

A 24 year old male presented with a gradual onset of gait problems, slurring of speech, and falls. Upon examination he had dysarthria with scanning speech, spasticity of all four limbs, a wide based gait, and hyporeflexia. His sister had similar symptoms. An MRI was performed (Fig. 5.4).

Explanation and Diagnosis

Figure 5.4 shows some generalized cerebral atrophy with marked cerebellar and pontine atrophy. The patient was diagnosed with spinocerebellar ataxia type 2 through genetic testing.

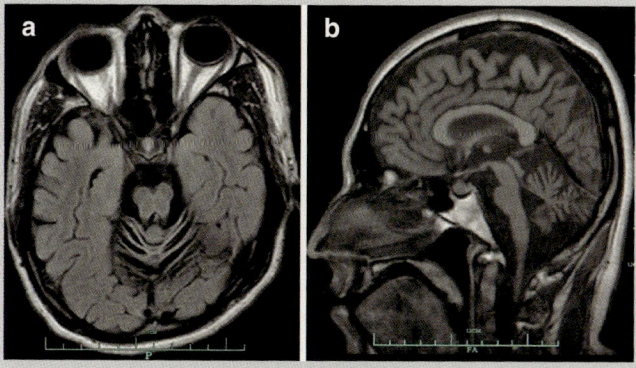

FIGURE 5.4 Axial FLAIR (**a**) and sagittal T1-weighted (**b**) MRI showing marked pontine and cerebellar atrophy

Case 5.5 Multiple Systems Atrophy
A 54 year old right handed male presented with a 3 years history of balance problems with falls. Additionally he had sexual dysfunction and postural dizziness. His systolic blood pressure would drop by 40 mmHg upon assuming an upright position after being supine. He had mild dysarthria with scanning speech and had mild features of Parkinsonism with bradykinesia and rigidity. An MRI was performed (Fig. 5.5).

Explanation and Diagnosis
Figure 5.5 shows generalized cerebral and marked cerebellar atrophy. The patient was diagnosed with multiple systems atrophy (MSA).

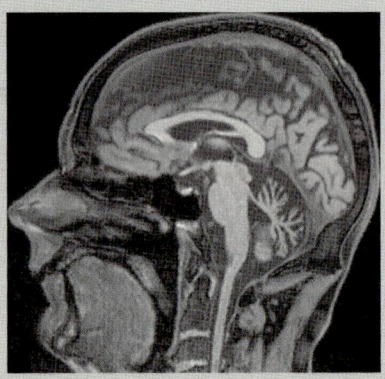

FIGURE 5.5 Sagittal T1-weighted MRI showing marked cerebellar atrophy

Case 5.6 Hummingbird Sign

A 64 year old male presented with a 2 year history of progressive left arm rigidity, falls, and Parkinsonism. On exam, he had evidence a supranuclear gaze palsy. An MRI was performed (Fig. 5.6)

Explanation and Diagnosis

This patient had a Parkinson plus syndrome with vertical gaze palsy and severe midbrain atrophy. Figure 5.6 shows a hummingbird sign which is often associated with progressive supranuclear palsy. In this case, the asymmetric presentation and asymmetric cerebral peduncles (the right is smaller, correlating with the left sided symptoms) makes the diagnosis corticobasal degeneration.

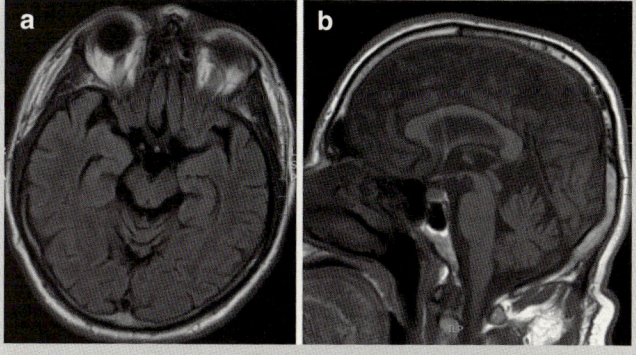

FIGURE 5.6 Axial FLAIR (a) and sagittal T1-weighted (b) MRI showing the hummingbird sign of severe midbrain atrophy with asymmetrical peduncle atrophy

Case 5.7 Spinal Muscular Atrophy

A 42 year old male presented with dysphagia after many years of gradually progressive weakness leading to an inability to walk. On exam there was significant atrophy and weakness of arms and legs with fasciculations and absent reflexes. An MRI was performed (Fig. 5.7).

Explanation and Diagnosis

Figure 5.7 shows extreme atrophy of the spinal cord with a relatively preserved cerebellum and cerebral hemispheres. The diagnosis was spinal muscular atrophy.

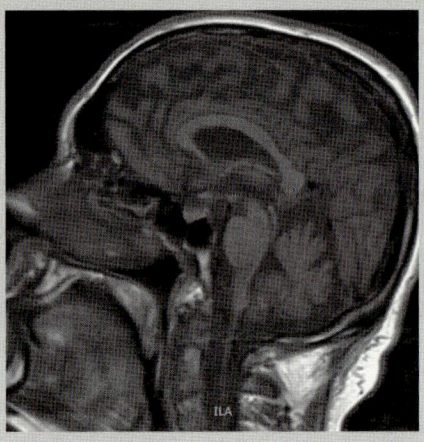

FIGURE 5.7 Sagittal T1-weighted MRI showing extreme spinal cord atrophy

Case 5.8 Creutzfeldt Jakob Disease

A 65 year old female presented with a 2 month history of confusion and ataxia. On exam she was found to have Gerstmann syndrome (agraphia, acalculia, right-left disorientation, finger agnosia), Wernicke aphasia, as well as ataxia and startle myoclonus. An MRI was performed (Fig. 5.8).

Explanation and Diagnosis

This is a case of rapidly progressive dementia with ataxia and myoclonus. Figure 5.8 shows the classic findings of Creutzfeldt Jakob disease, that of hyperintense FLAIR and restricted diffusion signal in the basal ganglia and/or cortical ribbon. The diffusion changes are often subtle and can be missed.

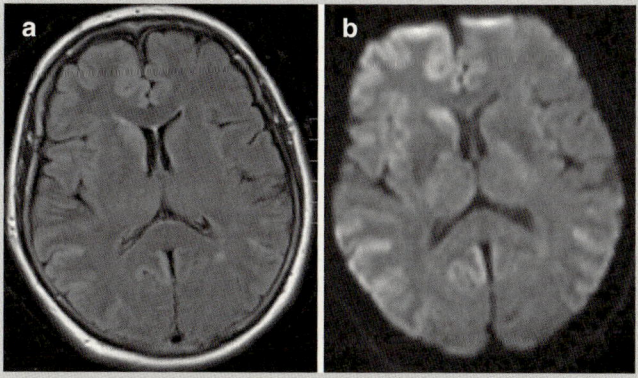

FIGURE 5.8 Axial FLAIR (**a**) and DWI (**b**) showing hyperintensity and restricted diffusion in the right caudate and cortical ribboning in the right frontal lobe, insula, medial occipital lobe and bilateral lateral occipital lobes

Chapter 6
Developmental Anomalies

Abstract   During the development of the nervous system, a number of things can go wrong, leading to a variety of developmental anomalies. Some of these are symptomatic from birth and can affect further development and functioning. Others may be asymptomatic or have more subtle effects which do not present until later in life. In this chapter we present several types of structural and developmental anomalies, including Arnold Chiari malformations, Dandy Walker malformation, tuberous sclerosis, mesial temporal sclerosis, arachnoid cysts and Rathke cleft cyst.

A.Q. Rana et al., *Neuroradiology in Clinical Practice*,
DOI 10.1007/978-3-319-01002-1_6,
© Springer International Publishing Switzerland 2013

Case 6.1 Arnold Chiari Malformation with Syrinx

A 34 year old male presented with numbness of finger tips and lower extremities. He also had headaches associated with coughing. On examination there was hyperreflexia of the lower extremities, bilateral unsustained clonus, equivocal planter responses, and decreased pinprick sensation in the C5 and C6 dermatomes. An MRI was performed (Fig. 6.1).

Explanation and Diagnosis

Figure 6.1 shows herniation of the cerebellar tonsils 2 cm below the foramen magnum and syrinx formation within the spinal cord extending from C2 to C6. These findings are consistent with Arnold Chiari malformation with syringomyelia.

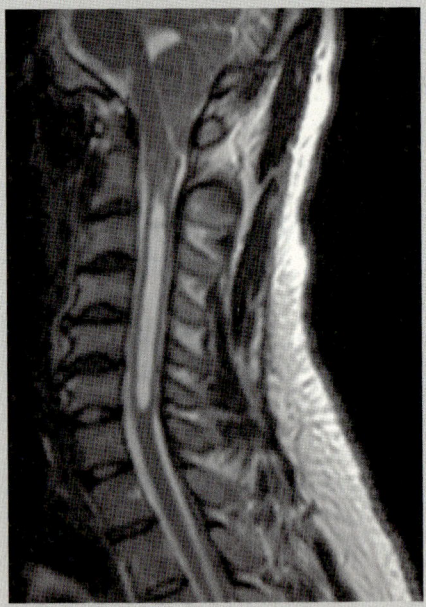

FIGURE 6.1 Sagittal T2-weighted MRI showing herniation of cerebellar tonsils and syrinx formation within the spinal cord

Case 6.2 Arnold Chiari Malformation with Disc Herniation

A 35 year old right-handed female presented with a long standing history of intermittent occipital headaches exacerbated by coughing, sneezing and straining. She also experienced episodes of neck pain without any radicular features. An MRI was performed (Fig. 6.2).

Explanation and Diagnosis

Figure 6.2 shows moderate cerebellar tonsillar herniation of approximately 8 mm with crowding of the foramen magnum. The patient was diagnosed with Arnold-Chiari type I malformation in addition to a C5/C6 disc herniation.

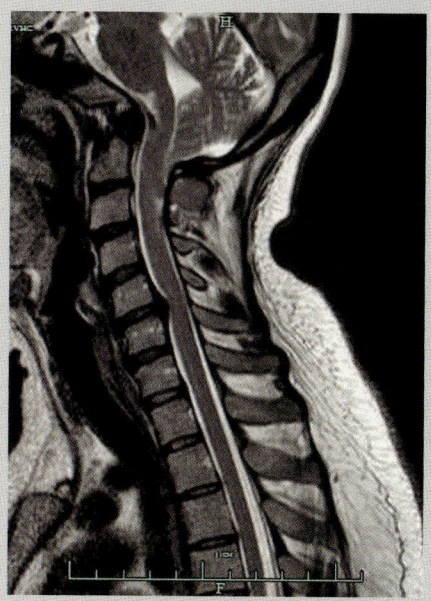

FIGURE 6.2 Sagittal T2-weighted MRI showing moderate cerebellar tonsillar herniation and C5-6 disc herniation

Case 6.3 Dandy-Walker Malformation
A 68 year old female presented with a long standing history of balance problems and falls. Upon examination she had wide based gait with mild slowness in walking speed. An MRI was performed (Fig. 6.3).

Explanation and Diagnosis
Figure 6.3 shows a small incompletely developed cerebellum a with wide cystic cerebrospinal fluid space in posterior cranial fossa. The patient was diagnosed with Dandy-Walker malformation.

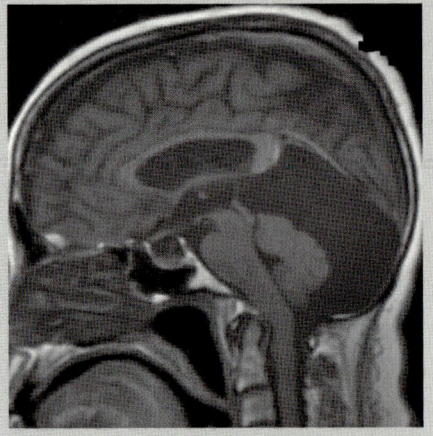

FIGURE 6.3 Sagittal T1-weighted MRI showing a Dandy-Walker malformation

Case 6.4 Mesial Temporal Sclerosis
A 27 year old right-handed male presented with a sudden onset of stiffness of both arms, with episodes of shaking of both sides of the body along with a loss of consciousness, tounge biting, and uninary incontinence. Each episode would last several minutes. An MRI was performed (Fig. 6.4).

Explanation and Diagnosis
Figure 6.4 shows a loss of volume of the left mesial temporal lobe, consistent with mesial temporal sclerosis, the likely source of this patient's seizure.

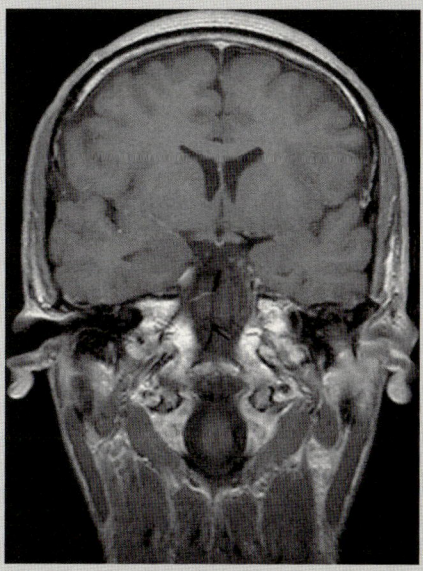

FIGURE 6.4 Coronal T1-weighted MRI showing left mesial temporal sclerosis

Case 6.5 Tuberous Sclerosis
A 32 year old patient with history of seizure disorder, encephalopathy, autism and behavioural issues was admitted after a seizure episode lasting 5 min. On exam, he had a rash of reddish spots (facial angiofibromas) on the nose and cheeks in a butterfly distribution. A CT scan was performed (Fig. 6.5).

Explanation and Diagnosis
Figure 6.5 shows the classical findings of tuberous sclerosis: cortical tubers and sub-ependymal nodules. Giant cell astrocytomas can also occur. Patients classically have facial angiofibromas in a butterfly pattern.

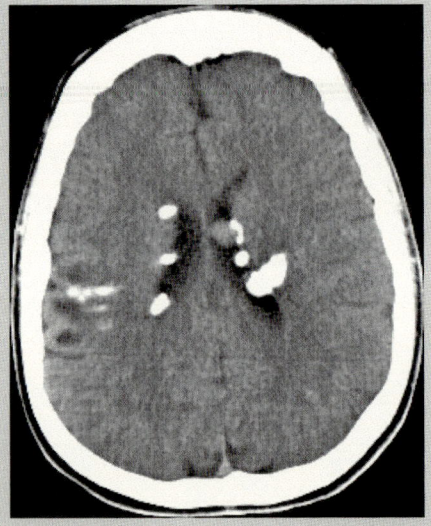

FIGURE 6.5 Axial CT showing numerous calcifications and a 1 cm soft tissue nodule associated with the ependymal calcification in the left lateral ventricle

Case 6.6 Arachnoid Cyst

A 32 year old male was referred for chronic headaches described as a "pressure wave sensation" in his head, occasional head fullness and light headedness, as well as intermittent visual dimming and obscuration. A CT was performed (Fig. 6.6).

Explanation and Diagnosis

Figure 6.6 shows a hypodense extraaxial mass in the left posterior fossa. This is an arachnoid cyst which was likely present from an early age.

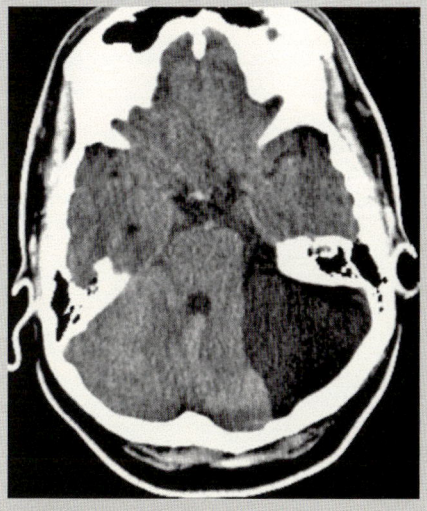

FIGURE 6.6 Axial CT showing hypodense wedge shaped lesion involving the left posterior fossa

Case 6.7 Rathke's Cleft Cyst

A 31 year old female was referred for new onset migraine headaches. The neurological exam was unremarkable. An MRI of the brain was performed (Fig. 6.7).

Explanation and Diagnosis

Figure 6.7 shows a hyperintense signal in the sella adjacent to the pituitary gland. This most likely represents a benign Rathke's cleft cyst and is unrelated to the headache presentation. Another condition that can occur in this region and be a cause of headache is pituitary haemorrhage seen with adenomas.

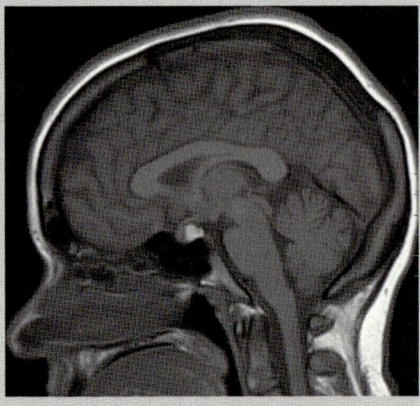

FIGURE 6.7 Sagittal T1 MRI showing a probable Rathke's cleft cyst in the sella

Chapter 7
Acquired/Structural Problems

Abstract With age, many structural problems arise from degenerative disease of the vertebral bodies. These can lead to disc herniations or spinal stenosis with varying degrees of nerve root or spinal cord compression. Other structural problems within the nervous system can involve the accumulation of cerebrospinal fluid in the brain. Depending on how this fluid accumulates, it may be asymptomatic or life threatening. In this chapter we present examples of degenerative spine disease leading to disc herniation or spinal stenosis, and fluid accumulations which cause hydrocephalus.

A.Q. Rana et al., *Neuroradiology in Clinical Practice*, 69
DOI 10.1007/978-3-319-01002-1_7,
© Springer International Publishing Switzerland 2013

Case 7.1 Spinal Stenosis
A 68 year old right-handed male presented with a history of neck pain and tingling of the hands which started 3 years ago and worsened with time. The neck pain was aggravated with physical activity. He had no weakness, bowel or bladder symptoms. An MRI was performed (Fig. 7.1).

Explanation and Diagnosis
Figure 7.1 shows degenerative changes in vertebral bodies C4-6 with osteophytes and small disc herniations leading to mild compression of thecal sac with myelopathic changes of spinal cord, consistent with spinal stenosis with cervical myelopathy.

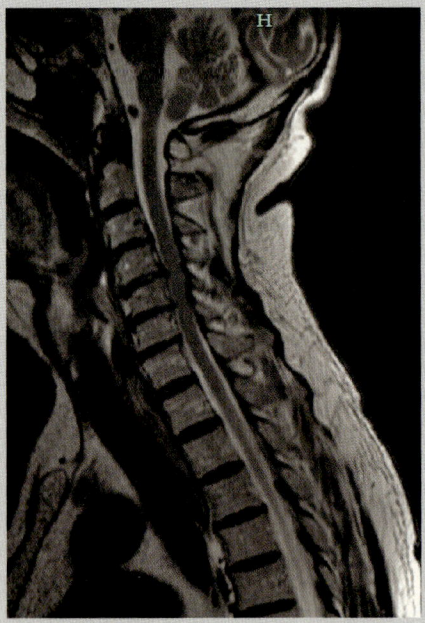

FIGURE 7.1 Sagittal T2-weighted MRI showing cervical stenosis

Case 7.2 Disc Herniation

A 48 year old right-handed female presented with neck pain radiating to her left upper extremity for almost 4 months after a motor vehicle accident. There was no head injury or loss of consciousness. She was taking over-the-counter analgesics but there was no significant improvement in her pain. Upon examination there was no focal weakness, sensory symptoms or trouble with bowel and bladder control. An MRI was performed (Fig. 7.2).

Explanation and Diagnosis

Figure 7.2 shows a large central disc herniation at C4/C5 with significant compression of the anterior aspect of the thecal sac and mild spinal cord compression.

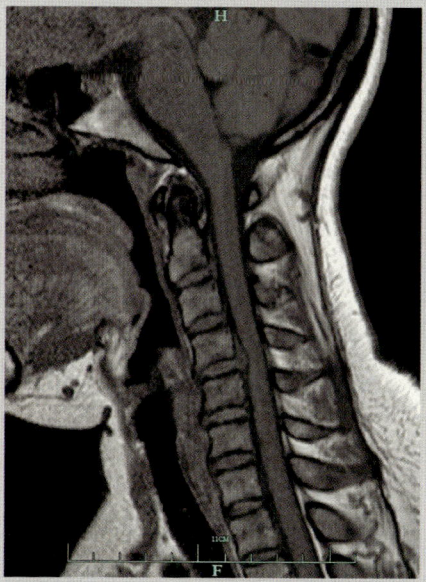

FIGURE 7.2 Sagittal T1-weighted MRI showing C4/5 disc herniation

Case 7.3 Non-communicating Hydrocephalus

A 25 year old left-handed male presented with complaints of "feeling pressure" in his head and early morning headaches. The headaches were intermittent and occurred on most days and lasted for several hours. They were moderate in intensity, exacerbated by supine positioning and were associated with nausea. Physical examination was unremarkable. A CT scan was performed (Fig. 7.3).

Explanation and Diagnosis

Figure 7.3 shows marked dilation of the lateral ventricles and loss of brain sulci consistent with non-communicating hydrocephalus and raised intracranial pressure.

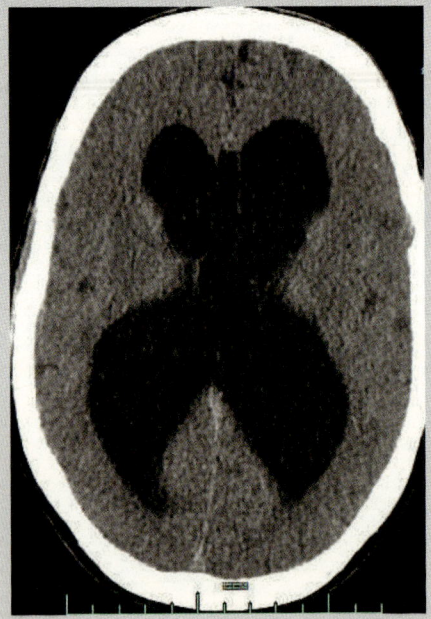

FIGURE 7.3 Axial CT showing marked dilatation of the lateral ventricles

Chapter 8
Neurotrauma

Abstract Rapid neuroimaging with CT scan is often used in trauma cases associated with altered level of consciousness as it can quickly reveal surgical emergencies such as fractures and bleeds. In this chapter we present cases of epidural and subdural hematomas, intracerebral contusions, cerebral edema with herniation and vertebral body fractures. Many of these are neurosurgical emergencies and require accurate and rapid assessment.

A.Q. Rana et al., *Neuroradiology in Clinical Practice*,
DOI 10.1007/978-3-319-01002-1_8,
© Springer International Publishing Switzerland 2013

Case 8.1 Epidural Hematoma

A 53 year old male presented with a history of falls and decreased level of consciousness. A CT scan was performed (Fig. 8.1).

Explanation and Diagnosis

Figure 8.1 shows a bi-convex hyperdensity in right frontal area with mild mass effect and midline shift. The correct diagnosis is acute right frontal epidural hematoma. This is a surgical emergency.

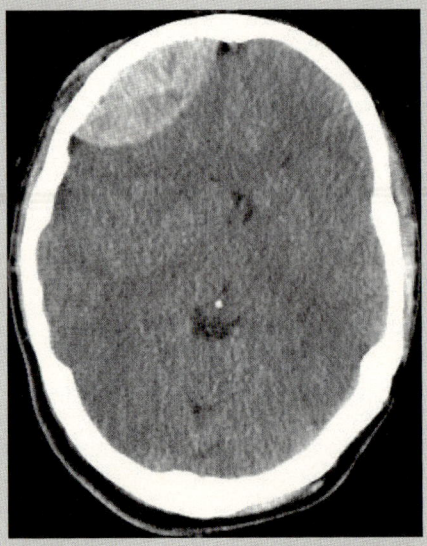

FIGURE 8.1   Axial CT showing right frontal epidural hematoma

Case 8.2 Subdural Hematoma
A 74 year old right-handed male presented after a fall on his driveway. He had consumed alcohol prior to the fall. He was noticed to have twitching of his right side which lasted for several seconds. A few hours later he had another episode of shaking of his right side lasting 30–60 s. A CT scan was performed (Fig. 8.2).

Explanation and Diagnosis
Figure 8.2 shows a concave hyperdensity over the left frontal and parietal areas, consistent with an acute subdural hematoma with mass effect and mild midline shift. Note the loss of the occipital horn due to mass effect. This is a surgical emergency.

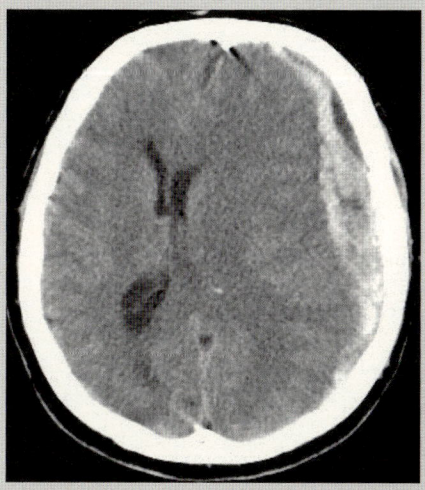

FIGURE 8.2 Axial CT showing left frontoparietal subdural hematoma with midline shift with loss of occipital horn

Case 8.3 Acute and Chronic Subdural Hematomas

A 73 year old male with a history of falls presented to the hospital with a decreased level of consciousness. A CT scan was performed (Fig. 8.3).

Explanation and Diagnosis

Figure 8.3 shows hyperdensities over the right frontal lobe and between the hemispheres, consistent with traumatic subdural hematomas due to falls. The hypodensity overlying the left frontal lobe is an old subdural hematoma likely secondary to previous head injury.

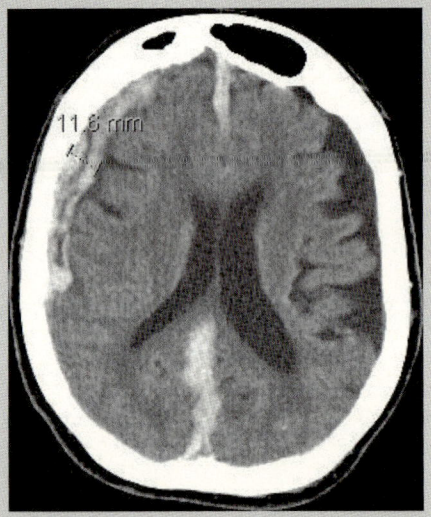

FIGURE 8.3 Axial CT showing acute right frontal subdural and inter-hemispheric hematoma, and a left frontal subdural hygroma

Case 8.4 Contusions

A 76 year old male who was on warfarin for atrial fibrillation experienced a fall without loss of consciousness. His heart rate was found to be 30 bpm. He hit his head on the ground and had a non-displaced occipital skull fracture. He was slightly confused and had headaches but no nausea, vomiting or any focal deficits. Serial CT scans were performed (Fig. 8.4).

Explanation and Diagnosis

Figure 8.4a shows very small hyperdense lesions involving both frontal lobes with parafalcine subdural hematoma and minor subarachnoid haemorrhage. Figure 8.4b shows significant evolution of both frontal lobe hyperdensities, with parafalcine subdural hematoma and minor subarachnoid haemorrhage. The diagnosis is traumatic intracerebral haemorrhage, with minor subdural and subarachnoid haemorrhage.

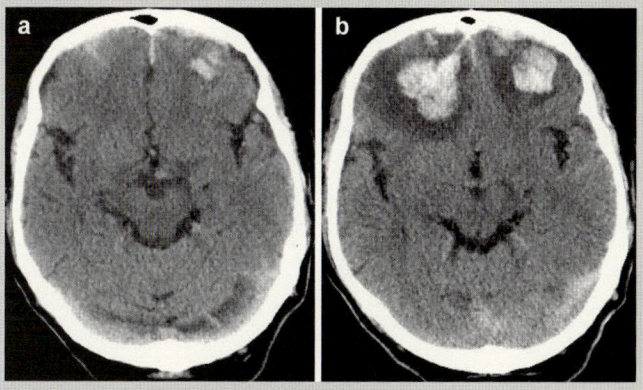

Figure 8.4 Axial CT on day 1 (a) and day 2 (b) showing hyperdense contusions and edema of both frontal lobes

Case 8.5 Cerebral Edema and Herniation

A 25 year old right-handed male fell down a flight of stairs while intoxicated. The patient had a mild headache with drowsiness but went to bed without seeking medical attention. The next morning he was unable to awaken and thus was admitted to hospital approximately 8 h after the fall.

He was unresponsive to verbal stimuli. He was only minimally moving his limbs to painful stimuli. His pupils were round, 3 mm in size, without any reaction to light. Motor testing showed normal tone and there was no preferential movement of any side more than the other. Deep tendon reflexes were absent. Plantar stimulation showed extensor responses on both sides. GCS was 5/15. CT scans were performed (Fig. 8.5).

Explanation and Diagnosis

Figure 8.5 shows a coup-contra coup injury pattern with left posterior tissue swelling and right frontal contusions. The patient underwent decompression craniotomies within 6 h of admission, however did not survive and died 48 h later.

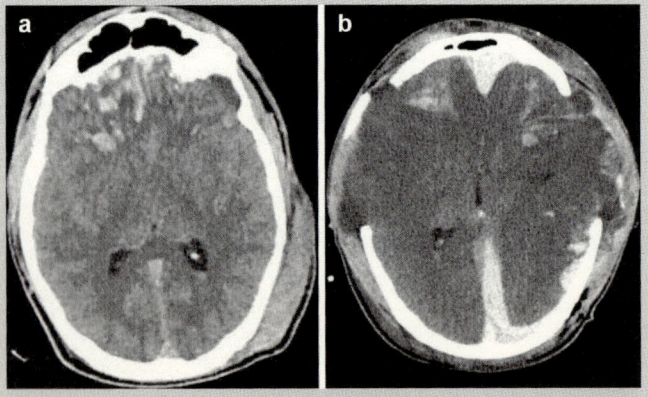

FIGURE 8.5 Axial CT showing extracranial soft tissue swelling, diffuse cerebral edema with sulcal effacement and intraparenchymal, haemorrhage before (**a**) and after (**b**) decompression craniotomies

Case 8.6 Vertebral Fracture

A 74 year old female presented with backache after a fall. Upon examination she displayed weakness of lower extremities, hyperreflexia, bilateral extensor planter responses and a sensory level up to T12. A CT scan was performed (Fig. 8.6).

Explanation and Diagnosis

Figure 8.6 shows a burst fracture of the T12 vertebral body with secondary spinal cord compression secondary

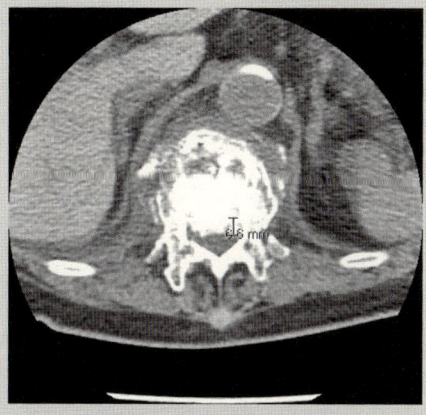

FIGURE 8.6 Axial spine CT showing a fracture of the T12 vertebral body

Chapter 9
Infectious Diseases

Abstract Many types of infectious organisms can affect the nervous system, including bacteria, fungi, viruses and parasites. It is beyond the scope of this reference manual to include every possible infection, but we include a description of imaging findings that are typical for tropical neurological diseases such as cerebral malaria, microsporidiosis, trypanosomiasis, leshmaniasis, dengue fever and snake bite. In addition, we present cases of CMV pachygyria, tuberculosis of the spine (Pott's disease) and spinal cord (syrinx), and complications of HIV infection such as toxoplasmosis and variable presentations of progressive multifocal leukodystrophy from JC virus.

A review of tropical neurological disease imaging characteristics.
Cerebral malaria: multiple cortical/subcortical contrast enhancing lesions with transtentorial herniation in fatal cases
Microsporidiosis: multiple ring enhancing lesions at the gray/white junction
African trypanosomiasis: basal ganglia hypodensities
CNS leshmaniasis: basal skull and meningeal inflammatory changes, optic nerve involvement, in addition to the more common signs and symptoms of peripheral neuropathy
Dengue fever: intracranial hemorrhage
Snake bite: hemorrhagic and ischemic infarct due to disseminated intravascular coagulation and toxin induced vasculitis

A.Q. Rana et al., *Neuroradiology in Clinical Practice*,
DOI 10.1007/978-3-319-01002-1_9,
© Springer International Publishing Switzerland 2013

Case 9.1 CMV Pachygyria
A neonate was found to have poor muscle tone (hypotonia), poor muscle control, feeding difficulties, small head circumference and new onset infantile spasms. TORCH panel showed CMV infection. A CT was performed (Fig. 9.1)

Explanation and Diagnosis
This neonate's hypotonia, feeding difficulties and poor muscle control as well as new onset infantile spasms can be attributed to intrauterine CMV infection as demonstrated by the TORCH panel. Figure 9.1 shows thickened cerebral cortices with few large gyri with incomplete development of the Sylvian fissures, consistent with pachygyria, a rare developmental disorder resulting from the abnormal migration of neurons in the developing brain and nervous system. This can be seen in other metabolic disorders such as Zellweger syndrome (peroxisome biogenesis disorder).

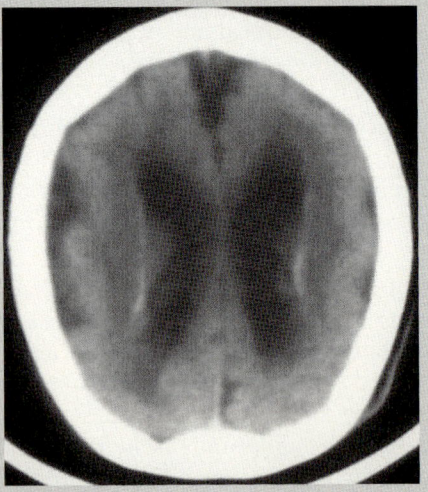

FIGURE 9.1 Axial CT showing pachygyria and incomplete development of the Sylvian fissures (Image courtesy of M. Koby)

Case 9.2 Pott's Disease

A 50 year old man with a history of recent travel abroad was admitted with sudden onset paraplegia and a several week history of fatigue, fever, malaise, night sweats, radiating low thoracolumbar pain and dysesthesia in the left leg. Extensive clinical and lab work up showed a significantly elevated ESR as well as positive skin PPD (tuberculin) test. A MRI spine was performed (Fig. 9.2).

Explanation and Diagnosis

Figure 9.2 shows lesions involving two vertebral bodies, with extensive destruction and erosion of the intravertebral space, leading to vertebral body collapse and spinal cord compression. A chest Xray showed multiple pulmonary nodules which were consistent with tuberculosis. The diagnosis was Pott's disease.

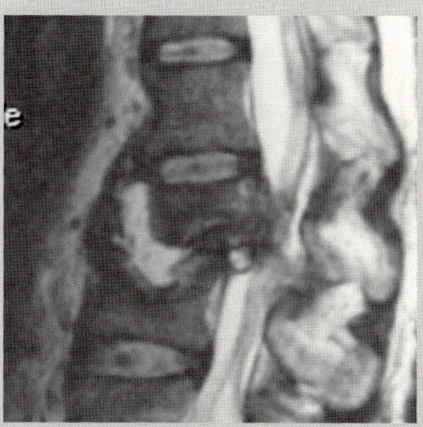

FIGURE 9.2 Sagittal T2-weighted MRI showing an extensively destructive lesion involving L1 and L2 vertebrae (Image courtesy of M. Koby)

Case 9.3 Tubercular Syrinx
A 35 year old right-handed female presented with lower limb paraparesis. She had a past history of pulmonary tuberculosis and tubercular meningitis which was managed with triple drug therapy for 6 months. An MRI of the spine was performed (Fig. 9.3).

Explanation and Diagnosis
Figure 9.3 shows an extensive hyperintense intramedullary signal within the spinal cord extending from C2 to the conus medullaris. The diagnosis is tubercular spinal cord syrinx.

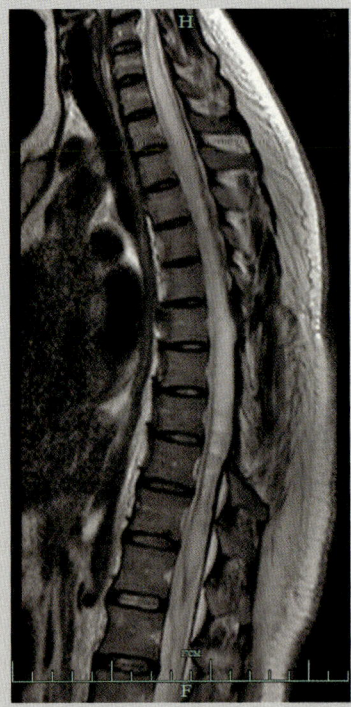

FIGURE 9.3 Sagittal T2-weighted MRI showing spinal cord syrinx

Case 9.4 Toxoplasmosis

A 55 year old male, HIV positive, was admitted for a 2 week history of left occipital headaches, dizziness, malaise, fever and occasional nausea and vomiting. An MRI was performed (Fig. 9.4).

Explanation and Diagnosis

Figure 9.4 shows circumscribed near spherical lesions surrounded by extensive vasogenic edema involving the left occipital lobe and basal ganglia. Edema also surrounds a cystic lesion in right basal ganglia. There is minimal midline shift. The clinical history and imaging is consistent with toxoplasmosis, which was confirmed by serology.

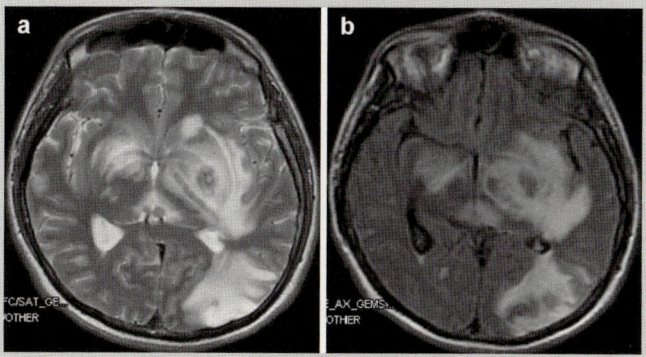

FIGURE 9.4 Axial T2-weighted (**a**) and FLAIR (**b**) MRI showing toxoplasmosis infection of the left occipital lobe and basal ganglia. There is minimal midline shift

Case 9.5 Progressive Multifocal Leukoencephalopathy – Confluent

A 49 year old male with HIV who was not on HAART therapy was admitted for subacute right hemiparesis and a subsequent fall. An MRI was performed (Fig. 9.5).

Explanation and Diagnosis

Figure 9.5 shows hyperintense signal in the white matter involving the left frontal and parietal lobes extending to the basal ganglia and the splenium of the corpus callosum. Given the clinical history and rapid progression the most likely diagnosis is progressive multifocal leukoencephalopathy (PML) caused by the JC virus in immunocompromised patients.

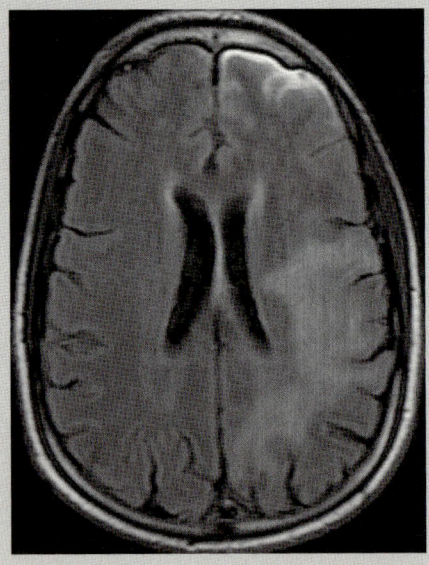

FIGURE 9.5 Axial FLAIR MRI showing left hemisphere confluent white matter hyperintensities

Case 9.6 Progressive Multifocal Leukoencephalopathy – Patchy

A 55 year old male with HIV presented with headache and encephalopathy with rapid clinical deterioration. An MRI was performed (Fig. 9.6).

Explanation and Diagnosis

Figure 9.6 shows hyperintense signals in the white matter of both hemispheres in a patchy distribution. Given the clinical history and rapid progression the most likely diagnosis is progressive multifocal leukoencephalopathy (PML) caused by the JC virus.

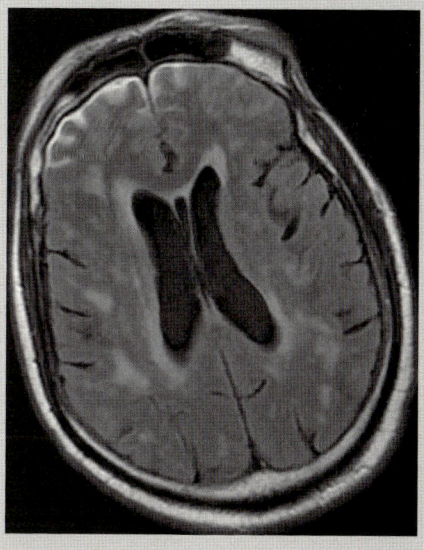

FIGURE 9.6 Axial FLAIR MRI showing bihemispheric multifocal confluent white matter hyperintensities

Chapter 10
Metabolic Disorders

Abstract A number of metabolic conditions can cause neurological symptoms, although not all are associated with imaging findings. It is important to know what imaging findings are significant and which are incidental. In this chapter we present incidental benign findings of basal ganglia calcification as well as the more serious central pontine myelinolysis which occurs with rapid correction of hyponatremia.

A.Q. Rana et al., *Neuroradiology in Clinical Practice*,
DOI 10.1007/978-3-319-01002-1_10,
© Springer International Publishing Switzerland 2013

Case 10.1 Basal Ganglia Calcification

A 63 year old right-handed female presented with a history of headaches. The neurological examination was unremarkable. She was diagnosed with tension headaches. A CT scan of head was done to rule out any secondary cause of headaches (Fig. 10.1).

Explanation and Diagnosis

Figure 10.1 shows hyper densities in the basal ganglia consistent with incidental calcification which is benign and is not a cause of headaches.

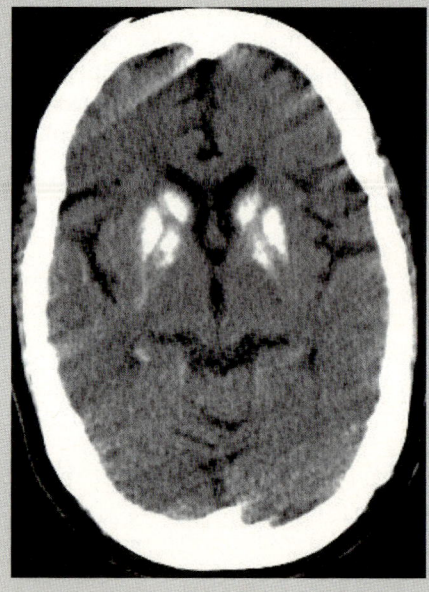

FIGURE 10.1 Axial CT showing bilateral basal ganglia calcification

Case 10.2 Central Pontine Myelinolysis

A 67 year old male with a history of alcohol use presented to the hospital in a drowsy state. His serum sodium level was 118 mmol/L. He was admitted to the hospital, and his serum sodium level was corrected to 135 mmol/L over 48 h. He developed quadriplegia. An MRI of the brain was performed (Fig. 10.2).

Explanation and Diagnosis

Figure 10.2 shows a large T2 hyperintense and T1 hypointense lesion in the pons consistent with central pontine myelinolysis (CPM), which occurred after rapid correction of the sodium and which was the cause of quadriplegia.

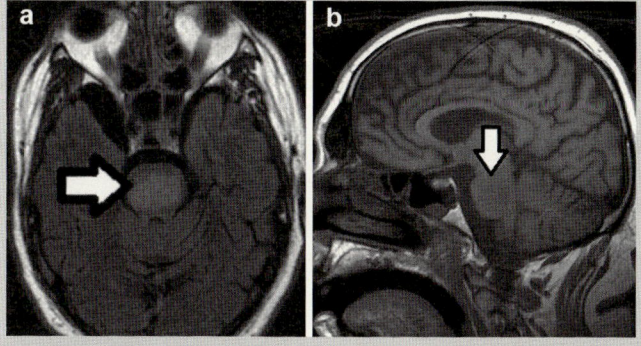

FIGURE 10.2 Axial FLAIR (**a**) and sagittal T1-weighted (**b**) MRI showing central pontine demyelination (*arrows*)

Chapter 11
Blood Vessel Imaging

Abstract Imaging of the blood vessel lumen can be best achieved by injecting a dye into the vessel and then imaging the dye with Xray, CT, or MR technologies, but a lot of information can be gleaned by measuring flow through the vessels with ultrasound. Because of the increased risk of stroke with conventional angiography, CT angiography or MR angiography is often the first choice of investigation for imaging intracranial arteries, but doppler ultrasound is still frequently used to assess the carotid arteries. Interpreting the results from any modality requires a good knowledge of vessel anatomy. In this chapter we present a quick review of the anatomy of the circle of Willis and provide case examples of vessel stenosis and aneurysms using MRA, CTA, and doppler ultrasound.

A.Q. Rana et al., *Neuroradiology in Clinical Practice*,
DOI 10.1007/978-3-319-01002-1_11,
© Springer International Publishing Switzerland 2013

Case 11.1 Anatomical Review

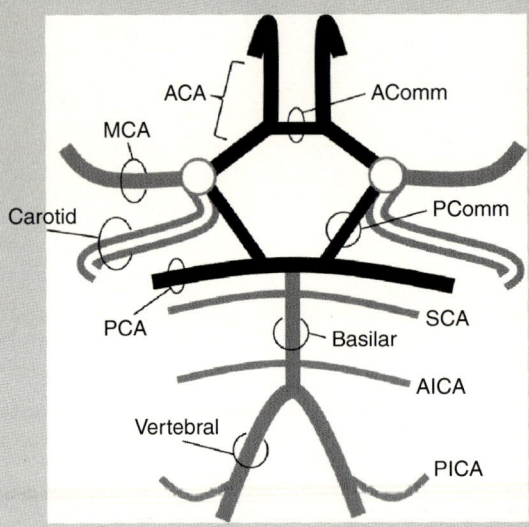

FIGURE 11.1 Diagram of the Circle of Willis and major intracranial blood vessels. *ACA* anterior cerebral artery, *AComm* anterior communicating artery, *MCA* middle cerebral artery, *PComm* posterior communicating artery, *PCA* posterior cerebral artery, *SCA* superior cerebellar artery, *AICA* anterior inferior cerebellar artery, *PICA* posterior inferior cerebellar artery

Case 11.2 Aneurysm (MRA)

A 55 year old right-handed male with no past medical history presented with new onset headaches. His neurological examination was normal. CBC, ESR, CRP, were normal. A CT scan of the brain showed a questionable hypodensity in right semi-centrum ovali. An MRA of the head was performed (Fig. 11.2).

Explanation and Diagnosis

Figure 11.2 is a gadolinium MRA showing a left middle cerebral artery aneurysm. Note the normal variance of blood vessel anatomy also, with absent posterior communicating arteries bilaterally.

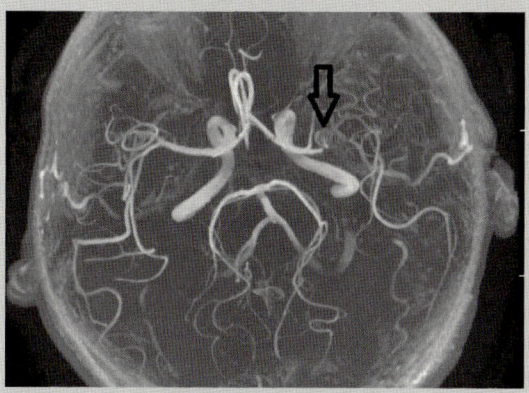

FIGURE 11.2 Axial view gadolinium MRA showing left middle cerebral artery aneurysm (*arrow*)

Case 11.3 MCA Occlusion (MRA)

An 81 year old right-handed female was admitted for acute onset of aphasia, right hemiparesis (face and arm greater than leg). Due to presentation out of the tPA window and due to possible hemorrhage on the admitting CT scan head, she was ineligible for tPA administration. She was admitted for stroke workup and management. An MRI showed a large acute-subacute, hemorrhagic infarct in the distribution of the left middle cerebral artery. An MRA was also performed (Fig. 11.3).

Explanation and Diagnosis

Figure 11.3 shows an occlusion of the left middle cerebral artery. Note that blood flow is not seen distally on the left. In addition, the right vertebral artery is not visualized and the left vertebral artery appears slightly irregular. Clinically the patient was able to be discharged to rehab in stable condition.

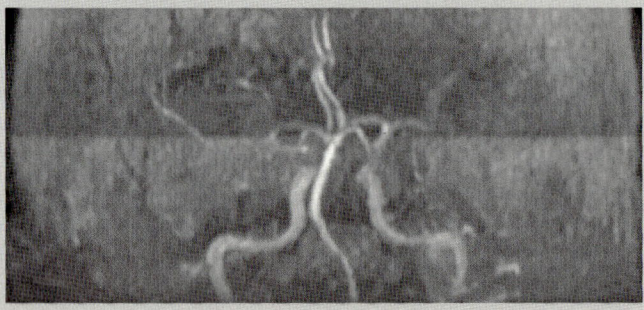

FIGURE 11.3 Coronal time of flight MRA showing left middle cerebral artery occlusion (seen on the right side of the image)

Case 11.4 Bilateral ICA Stenosis (CTA)

A 62 year old male presented with recurrent left sided weakness. An MRI of the brain revealed multiple small acute strokes in the right middle cerebral artery territory. A CTA was performed to look for a critical stenosis (Fig. 11.4).

Explanation and Diagnosis

Recurrent right hemisphere ischemia was likely secondary to significant disease (70–80 % stenosis) of the right internal carotid artery, as shown in Fig. 11.4.

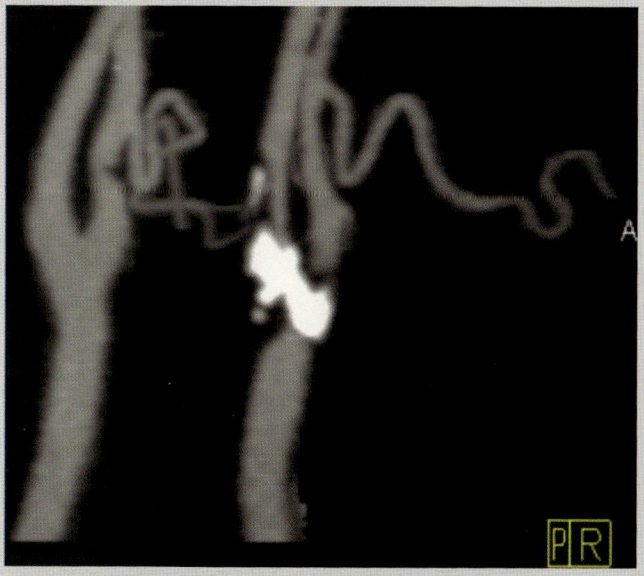

FIGURE 11.4 CTA of carotid arteries (rotated such that the left carotid is on the left in the image) showing patent left internal carotid with 50 % stenosis of the external carotid and calcification of the right carotid bulb with 70–80 % stenosis of the right internal carotid

Case 11.5 Internal Carotid Occlusion (Doppler Ultrasound)

A 60 year old male with multiple neurovascular risk factors was admitted for altered mental status and left hemisensory alterations. A CT revealed an acute left MCA territory stroke. A carotid ultrasound was performed (Fig. 11.5).

Explanation and Diagnosis

Figure 11.5 shows that there is no flow in the right ICA, consistent with total occlusion. Given the stroke presentation, this was the symptomatic carotid, but due to its 100 % occlusion, carotid endarterectomy is not required. The patient was discharged on antiplatelet agents.

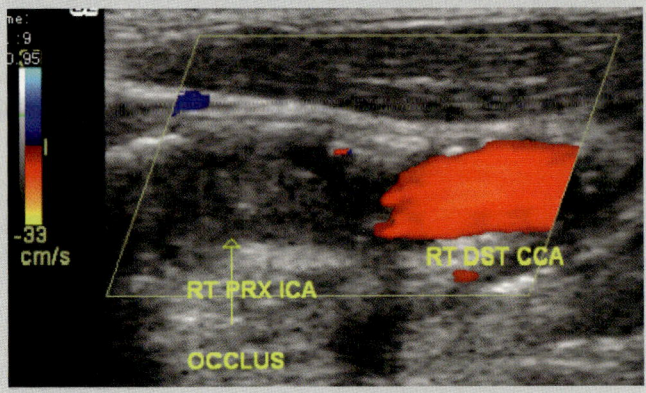

FIGURE 11.5 Carotid duplex ultrasound demonstrating complete occlusion of the right internal carotid artery (*ICA*) and 50–60 % stenosis of the right common carotid artery (*CCA*). Angle of insonation is 60°. The ICA is occluded by a noncalcified thrombus

Index

A.Q. Rana et al., *Neuroradiology in Clinical Practice*,
DOI 10.1007/978-3-319-01002-1,
© Springer International Publishing Switzerland 2013

Printed by Printforce, the Netherlands